Home and Community Care for Chronically Ill Children

Home and Community Care for Chronically Ill Children

James M. Perrin, M.D.

Associate Professor of Pediatrics
Harvard Medical School
Children's Service
Massachusetts General Hospital
Boston

May W. Shayne, M.S.W.

Research Associate
Institute for Public Policy Studies
Vanderbilt University
Nashville

Sheila R. Bloom, M.S.

Research Associate
General Pediatric Research Unit
Massachusetts General Hospital
Boston

New York   Oxford
OXFORD UNIVERSITY PRESS
1993

Oxford University Press

Oxford   New York   Toronto
Delhi   Bombay   Calcutta   Madras   Karachi
Kuala Lumpur   Singapore   Hong Kong   Tokyo
Nairobi   Dar es Salaam   Cape Town
Melbourne   Auckland   Madrid

and associated companies in
Berlin   Ibadan

Copyright © 1993 by Oxford University Press, Inc.

Published by Oxford University Press, Inc.,
200 Madison Avenue, New York, New York 10016

Oxford is a registered trademark of Oxford University Press

Library of Congress Cataloging-in-Publication Data
Perrin, James M. (James Marc)
Home and community care for chronically ill children /
James M. Perrin, May W. Shayne, Sheila R. Bloom.
p.   cm.   Includes bibliographical references and index.
ISBN 0-19-507120-4
1. Chronically ill children—Home care—United States.
2. Chronically ill children—Services for—United States.
I. Shayne, May W. II. Bloom, Sheila R. III. Title.
[DNLM: 1. Chronic Disease—in infancy & childhood.
2. Community Health Services.
3. Family—psychology. 4. Home Nursing—in infancy & childhood.
5. Quality of Health Care—economics.
WS 200 P458h]   RJ380.P47   1993
362.1′9892—dc20   DNLM/DLC
for Library of Congress   92–22536

9 8 7 6 5 4 3 2 1
Printed in the United States of America
on acid-free paper

Foreword

Julianne Beckett

I salute the efforts of Dr. Perrin, Ms. Shayne, and Ms. Bloom to bring the need for family-centered, community-based services for families and children to a broader audience of families, health professionals, educators, and public policymakers. They clearly describe the impact of home care on families with children with complex medical conditions, the service system that supports families, and the costs and quality of care, and they provide sound recommendations for improving this system.

The current political climate for children and families, for health care financing, and for people with disabilities holds great promise for future change along the lines proposed in this book. Politicians and policymakers have come to realize that support for all children and families must be forthcoming if the United States is to maintain its leadership role into the next century. Employers, health insurance executives, health care providers, workers, and politicians are alerted to the acute problems of our system in financing health care services and seem to be on the verge of addressing some longstanding inequities. A changing national view of disability led to recent legislation, the Americans with Disabilities Act, which opens doors to employment, recreation, accommodations, and other community programs that have long been closed to adults and children with disabilities. These three issues of family support, financing of care, and access, are crucial to the successful integration of our health-impaired youngsters into society, and are lucidly examined by the authors.

Society has begun to understand the potential of children with severe disabilities and what can be done to improve the lives of all children and their families in our communities. With this book we, as advocates for children with complex medical conditions and their families, will be better able to assess the current state of services for our youngsters and to analyze the effects of the evolving public policy agenda. As the parent of a child who is ventilator-assisted, as a former public school teacher, as a woman who has worked to make public policies and public institutions more responsive to families' needs, I well appreciate the importance of what the authors have undertaken and applaud their efforts.

Preface

Rapidly rising health care costs, large numbers of uninsured Americans, questions about the effectiveness and quality of care, and the growing need for long-term care for a rapidly increasing elderly population attract the attention of policymakers, insurers, employers, health care professionals, and consumers. These issues have helped to bring health care and long-term care to center stage in the public agenda. Most attention to children's health care issues has focused on unmet needs for prenatal and infant care or to special programs and needs of adolescent populations. Yet home care and long-term care for children also merit attention to improve the lives of children and their families. But society also will benefit by improving the long-term functioning of children with severe illness. Providing families high-quality health services greatly increases the likelihood that youngsters growing up in these families, despite severe illnesses, can become effective participants in adult society.

Most children are healthy and use relatively few health services, especially when compared to older age groups. Children with conditions such as cystic fibrosis, hemophilia, respiratory impairments requiring home and school ventilator support, complications of premature birth, leukemia, severe kidney disease, bronchopulmonary dysplasia, muscular dystrophy, spina bifida, and hundreds of other relatively rare and severe illnesses use a disproportionately large share of inpatient and outpatient child health care services.

With advances in medical technology and treatment, at least 90 percent of children with severe illnesses now survive to young adulthood and beyond. Thus, in addition to their heavy use of medical and surgical services, this group of children with chronic illnesses utilizes almost all long-term care among the young. Unlike the elderly, on whom public consideration of long-term care has focused, children are in the most rapid stage of development, with ever-changing emotional, social, and educational needs. And, most dra-

matically, in ever-growing numbers, the children live at home. Most children
with ventilators, respirators, and feeding tubes are no longer forced by dependence on technology to remain in the hospital. Their portable equipment
makes them sufficiently mobile to live with their families and to attend school
in their communities. Thus, youngsters with even the severest health conditions are increasingly visible in schools and communities. Services provided
in or near home, rather than in hospitals and other institutional settings, have
the potential both to improve the lives of children whose health conditions
require reliance on intensive, high-technology services, and to reduce the high
costs of hospital care.

The increased survival of children with severe illnesses and the growing
number who live at home create new demands on the health care, education,
and community services systems. The health care system, skilled at providing
care for episodes of acute illnesses, must make the adjustments necessary to
provide long-term care to children with chronic, complex conditions. Specialty care in hospitals must be integrated with primary care that is delivered in
local communities convenient to the children and their families. Home health
agencies, most often specializing in care of the elderly, must develop skills in
child development and family issues in their expanding pediatric practice.
Schools must find new ways to provide medications and adjust teaching to
frequent, illness-related absences for students who have more health-care
needs but the same academic potential as healthy children. Accustomed to
teaching children with developmental disabilities in special education programs, schools must now tailor their programs to youngsters with less familiar
and at times alarming illnesses. Community services and activities—Scouts
and recreation clubs—must work with families to integrate health-impaired
children into programs that are vital to their social development and self-
esteem.

Great though the challenge to health, education, and community services
may be, the challenge to families is greater. Parents are clear about who
should care for their ill children and where the children should live. They want
to raise their own children in their own homes, but the demands are formidable. Families face intense and unpredictable medical crises. Parents must
become expert in byzantine health insurance provisions and special education
laws and regulations. They must have technical skills to keep breathing and
feeding equipment functional. They must be diplomatic managers of home-
care nurses and aides, therapists, and medical and surgical specialists. They
must hold their jobs, often in order to keep their health insurance. They must
nurture their ill children, taking into account illness-related limitations while
providing the structure, discipline, and behavioral expectations and challenges

that all young people require. They must be sure that they do not neglect their other children and their own emotional needs, lest the family burn out.

Several programs in different parts of the country are leading the way in responding to the challenges of caring for children with severe chronic health conditions in their homes. To understand better the issues that the health and education systems, communities, and families face, our multidisciplinary team (pediatrician, social worker, and health administrator/analyst) visited and collected data on ten of these exemplary programs. We interviewed individuals who were involved in all aspects of home care—program managers, physicians, nurses, educators, insurers, occupational and physical therapists, care coordinators. Most telling were the visits with the families and children. We met them in program offices and in their homes, in New York City, in rural Iowa, in Chicago, and in small Florida towns. This book is an account of the families' cumulative experiences and an analysis of the issues that the experience embodies.

The book aims to lay common ground for all who have reason and responsibility to enhance the capability of families to care for their ill children over the long term at home. Families, professionals, and policymakers comprise the audience. Family advocates will find the book useful in setting agendas and identifying viable options. Educators and health providers, especially physicians, nurses, and home-care agency staff, will find guidance for program development. Maternal and child health leaders, education administrators, and state and federal legislative staffs, especially those examining high-risk insurance pools, comprehensive health insurance programs, and catastrophic care, will find information, analyses, and cogent suggestions for new directions in policies and programs.

This book is based mainly on the stories of families, told to us in many settings or shared indirectly from their writings, published or in letters. It is the families' stories that best define the issues and point the way to solutions. Several of the books' seven chapters begin with issues raised by families in our visits with them, and their comments and concerns weave throughout the text.

Chapter 1 describes the population of children in home care and three social trends that are propelling the issue of home care onto the public agenda: the rights of families, the growth of technology, and concern about containing the costs of medical care.

Chapter 2 describes the impact on families of assuming the responsibility of providing care at home to children with special health needs. The work of parents in caring for their child, their isolation and need for support, and the stress they experience are discussed here. Chapter 3 examines the organization and delivery of services. Issues concerning health services include the narrow range of services usually available, the lack of coordination of care, and problems in gaining access to services that families and children need. Problems in educational programs include the inappropriateness of special education for many health-impaired children and major gaps in developmental and vocational counseling.

Chapter 4 deals with the quality of care, distinguishing between technical and interpersonal aspects of care. The chapter defines criteria for assessing the quality of care within a framework of process, structure, and outcome measures. Chapters 5 and 6 deal with financial issues. In Chapter 5 we detail the financial cost to families of home care, including payments for nursing, social services, equipment, and home modifications and opportunity costs for families as well as the costs of medical and surgical services. The strengths and weaknesses of the major private and public programs that pay for care are detailed in Chapter 6.

The final chapter offers recommendations for national and state policy and for programs for care at home for chronically ill children and their families. Three principles undergird the recommendations: Families must be empowered to direct their children's care, families must have access to a flexible and broad range of services, and children and families must be integrated into the fabric of their communities. From these principles flow recommendations for changes in the organization and provision of services, quality assurance, and financing of care. As children with complex health conditions move from hospital to home in ever-increasing numbers, the challenge is to enable their families to care for them and to nurture their development. With adequate policies and programs in place, the children, their families, and the nation stand to realize the benefits of caring for children with chronic illnesses where they should live—at home.

Acknowledgments

This book reflects the efforts of many people. A distinguished National Advisory Committee met to review our work at various stages. Betsy Anderson, Thomas Boat, Tessie Cleveland, Steve Freedman, Debra Hymovich, Linda Randolph, and Ruth Stein drew upon their extensive experience and knowledge to provide invaluable guidance to the study. The manuscript benefitted greatly from readings by Julie Beckett, Henry Ireys, and John MacQueen. Our colleague Deborah Walker enriched our work with her insights and support. We are grateful to Linda Moynihan for her help in designing the study, to Kelly McBride for her fine secretarial and telephone support during the early phase of the study, and to Barbara Rich for her competent, patient skill in preparing the manuscript.

Funding for the study was provided by the Bureau of Maternal and Child Health of the U.S. Department of Health and Human Services, grants MCJ-473623 and MCJ-253795. We appreciate the leadership, counsel, and review from Vince Hutchins, Merle McPherson, and their colleagues in the Bureau of Maternal and Child Health.

We especially thank the parents and children, administrators, and providers at the program sites whom we interviewed. The study would have been impossible without their generosity, eloquence, and graciousness in sharing their experiences with us. We provide here the names of providers and program staff in appreciation of their time and special contribution to this work.

Child Health Specialty Clinics: Richard Nelson, Julie Beckett, Kathy Bowers, Milo Colton, Mickey Rook McDaniel, Dottie Doolittle, Trula Foughty, Josie Gittler, Cari Gordinier, Tom Hulme, Kathi Kellen, Helen Kueter, Susan Lagos, John MacQueen, Deb McClimon, Brenda Moore, Ann Riley, Phyllis Ruiz, Jay Van Dyke, James Ziska

Children's Memorial Hospital: Martha Fleming, Laura Frost, Candy Wilhite

Coordinating Center for Home and Community Based Care: Joanne Kaufman, Nancy Bond, Dianne Feeney, Edward Feinberg, Karen-Ann Lichtenstein, Barbara McCord, June McGuckian, Deeley Middleton, Priscilla Phillips, Debbie Ribakow, Alan Rosenblatt

COPE—CCICC Program: Florence Marshall

Division of Services for Crippled Children: Edward Lis, Eugene Bilotti, Lu Ann Aday, Marlene Aitken, Ron Andersen, Pat Craft, Lauri Ford, Dorothy Green, Donna Harris, Donna Hope, Renata Hornick, Noreen McAndrews Kolman, Kevin McMurtry, Colleen Monahan, Kathleen Murphy, Mark Splaingard

La Rabida Children's Hospital and Research Center: Arthur Kohrman, Javeed Akhter, Evelyn Allen, Eugene Bilotti, Susan Connell, Helen Emery, Neil Hochstadt, Ann Holman, Paula Jaudes, Noreen McAndrew Kilman, Mary Petrella, Sandy Scannell, Susan Sullivan-Bolyai, Frank Thorpe

Pediatric Home Care: Ruth Stein, Henry Adam, Eliot Barsh, Beverly Ellman, Laurie Gordon, Aida LiBasci, Sunni Levine, Mary McCort, Robert Ruben, Maris Rosenberg, Edna Sobel, Marlene Tappley, Robert Weiss

REACH: Steve Freedman, Patricia Pierce, Linda Pingatore, Lizzie Lenon, Daryl Mase, Gerold Schiebler

Regional Hemophilia Center, New York Hospital: Margaret Hilgartner, Jeanine Aquino, Laura Burdich, Thom Harrington, Lynne Jacobs, Elaine Kane, Judith Levi, Gilda Martoglio, Mimi Meyers

Visiting Nurse Service of New York: Marilyn Liota, Nancy Archer, Maureen D'Iorio, Mary Ho, Fay Hogg, Doreen Nelkin-Warantz, Lisa Martin, Carol Odnoha, Lucy Rodriguez, Debbie Saltzburg, Jeanne Sloan, Jackie Taubman.

Finally, we are ever cognizant of the vision of Nicholas Hobbs (1915–1983) who initiated our studies of policies affecting chronically ill children and their families over a decade ago. Nick first identified the issue of long-term illness in childhood, recognized the central dynamism of families in caring for chronically ill children, and focused on the community and environmental interactions with families. His remarkable leadership continues to guide many efforts for children and families.

This book has depended on the participation of all these colleagues and friends and their commitment to family-centered, community-based care. Errors of fact or judgment are, of course, ours, not theirs. We hope that our combined efforts will contribute to improved policies and programs that enable families to provide home care for children with severe health conditions.

Contents

Home and Community Care for Chronically Ill Children

1

Introduction

Jack George, a 15-year-old, has a severe progressive neuromuscular disease that first appeared almost a decade ago. Since then he has slowly lost most of his muscular ability. Now he is confined to bed, unable to care for himself, and with a tube in his throat (tracheostomy) to assist his breathing. His current medical status is fairly stable, yet his future is clouded as he progressively loses muscular function. He spends much of his time at home, either in his special bed or moving around in a wheelchair with other people's help. Like many other teenagers, Jack is intensely interested in his looks, in sex, in television programs, and in sports cars. Alert and outgoing, he makes people laugh with his never-flagging humor. His insight and sensitivity impress all who know him.

Jack's mother has two younger daughters; his father left the family when Jack was 9 and he has had no contact with his son in several years. Jack started kindergarten with other children his own age, but as his disease progressed and he missed school, he was less and less able to keep up. From age 9 to 12, he was more often out of school than in it, and he fell far behind his classmates. About three years ago, Jack's mother learned about a program that provided home nursing services through a large community hospital near her inner-city home. Since that time, although Jack's medical condition has slowly deteriorated, his and his family's life-style has clearly improved. Rather than traveling by ambulance and waiting in stark hospital corridors for checkups, the family has visits from a nurse who has become Jack's confidante and a friend and support for the family. He trusts the nurse who comes regularly to visit the family and, with her help, has been able to talk about the normal issues of adolescent turmoil as well as about the ways that his illness prevents him from doing many things other teens can do. The nurse has the professional skills to assess Jack's medical needs and discuss them with pediatric and specialty physicians. Through this connection, Jack's mother now feels she has a strong advocate in the system, someone who helps her not only by answering questions but also by helping her formulate them well. In the past, she spent much of her time traveling from appointment to appointment and trying to follow unclear, often contradictory, orders from health providers. Mrs. George now has greater responsibility for Jack's care, knows where to get advice and help, and feels more capable and responsible for the needs of her own family. The community hospital program also aided Mrs. George arrange home tutoring three times a week to help Jack catch up with his age-mates in math, English, and other subjects.

Philip Stevens has Goldenhar's syndrome, a congenital condition. Like many other congenital abnormalities, Goldenhar's syndrome is rare, and the physicians attending Philip's birth were unable to diagnose his condition for several months. He was born with eyes placed slightly to the sides and with his right ear incompletely developed and positioned farther back than usual. He also had a club foot. At a few months of age, it was apparent that his vision and hearing were severely impaired. Health providers gave Philip's parents conflicting information about his condition, what could be done for it, and what to expect from Philip as he matured. Now, two years later, his parents are still angry because the physicians did not communicate effectively, offered meager support, and provided little help in finding answers for their questions.

Both of Philip's parents are professionals, his mother a respiratory therapist and his father a lawyer. The family traveled hundreds of miles from home to talk with specialists about Philip's condition, to learn what they could about this rare problem, its treatment, and its outlook. With help from their pediatrician, they did most of the work themselves to seek out specialists and to find the answers to their questions.

Philip is home with his mother most of the time now. At age 2, he is a playful, mischievous boy. He wears thick glasses and a hearing aid to help compensate for his impairments. Like Jack, he has a tracheostomy and he is somewhat delayed in his speech as a result. He is learning to communicate by sign language and has begun to make understandable noises by occasionally closing his tracheostomy. Learning from the experience of other families of children with complex health conditions, Philip's parents now have some home-based services to help them care for Philip. A home health aide comes for two 4-hour shifts a week. Mrs. Stevens has little need for home nursing services, being very accomplished herself in providing her son's respiratory treatments and meeting his nursing care needs. What she does need is a homemaker, someone to free her from household tasks so that she can occasionally play with Philip in a relaxed way as a parent. But the family's health insurance covers only in-home health services; homemaker services aren't covered. The family lives in a community with a strong early intervention program. Through this program, Philip has a special teacher who comes to his home once a week and who has supplied learning tools and games to encourage Philip's development.

At first, most services that the Stevens family received were medical or surgical care for Philip's multiple conditions. From other parents, Mrs. Stevens learned the importance of other services for Philip and the family. After more than a year and a half of fighting for comprehensive services for her child, Mrs. Stevens now believes she knows what might work and feels more in control of the situation. She carries out the planning and decision making for Philip's health and home services, relying on her husband, other family advocates, her pediatrician, and one of the specialists for advice.

CHILDREN WHO REQUIRE HOME- AND COMMUNITY-BASED SERVICES

The two families we have described represent the growing number of families with children receiving increasingly complex and technologically sophisticated health services at home rather than in hospitals. This book details the background of home- and community-based care for chronically ill children, the problems and prospects for families, and potential solutions for a growing problem.

Many health conditions cause youngsters to need specialized equipment or specialized care at home. The term *technology dependent* has received much attention in recent years as a way of describing people who depend on complicated equipment to maintain body functions. Children who are dependent on technology form a small but growing part of a much larger spectrum of children with health conditions who may require specialized home- or community-based services.

Current estimates are that 15 million to 20 million American children have some kind of chronic health condition (Gortmaker & Sappenfield, 1984). Most of these conditions are mild or moderate in their impact on children, and relatively few require major ongoing attention at the home and community levels. Severe health conditions, ones that are likely to require extensive daily caretaking, affect between 1 million and 2 million youngsters (Newacheck, Budetti, & McManus, 1984) (Fig. 1–1). Many different conditions fit this category of severe illness, and examples are listed in Table 1–1. Children face a large number of different chronic health conditions that may cause severe impairment, although each individual condition (with few exceptions) is uncommon. Among the chronic physical health conditions that affect children, asthma is by far the most common, affecting approximately $2^1/2$ million youngsters in the United States. Most cases of asthma also are mild or moder-

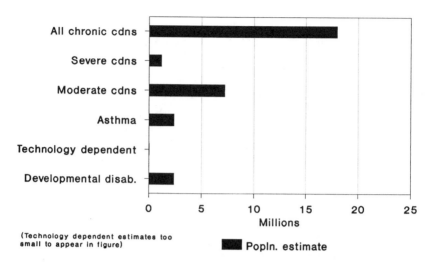

Figure 1-1. Estimated numbers of children with chronic health conditions or developmental disabilities, United States, 1988.

Table 1-1. Chronic Health Conditions Requiring Medical and Nursing Procedures at Home

Examples of childhood conditions	Special issues	Medical intensity in the home		
		High	Medium	Low
Hemophilia	Home clotting factor		✔	
Diabetes	Measurement of blood sugar, diet, insulin injections			✔
Thalassemia	Hospitalization for transfusions			✔
Ventilator-dependency	Major equipment at home	✔		
Short-bowel syndrome	Feeding or IV equipment	✔		
Cystic fibrosis	Home pulmonary treatment, diets		✔	
Spina bifida	Mobility equipment, urinary care		✔	
Muscular dystrophy	Wheelchairs, ventilators		✔	
Leukemia (and other cancers)	Protection from infection			✔
AIDS	Protection from infection, developmental effects			✔
Sickle cell anemia	Pain, prevention of crises			✔
Down syndrome	Developmental effects			✔
Congenital heart disease	Complicated medications, O_2 treatment		✔	
Arthritis	Wheelchair, physical therapy		✔	
Asthma	Home nebulization			✔

ate, and only about 10 percent of children with asthma have severe forms of the illness. However, asthma accounts for one-third to one-half of all *severe* childhood health conditions.

Children dependent on technology include those who require assisted ventilation to help their breathing, specialized feeding by intravenous (IV) tubes (parenteral nutrition), and IV antibiotics over a prolonged period. In 1987, the upper limit of estimates of the size of this population was 17,000 children (U.S. Congress, 1987) (Fig. 1–2). It thereby accounts for a very small percentage of the total number of children with severe illnesses. Table 1–1 lists examples of some of the childhood health conditions that require specialized home- and community-based services, along with examples of the specific issues that may relate to any one condition. This list provides a partial view of selected childhood health conditions and is not intended to be exhaustive.

WHY CARE AT HOME FOR SICK CHILDREN?

Three main forces have propelled the recent expansion of home-based services for severely ill children: greater awareness of the rights of families (Singer & Butler, 1987), technological advances improving survival of children and allowing more out of hospital treatments (Perrin, 1990; U.S. Department of Health and Human Services, 1982), and emphasis on cost containment in health care (Enthoven & Kronick, 1989).

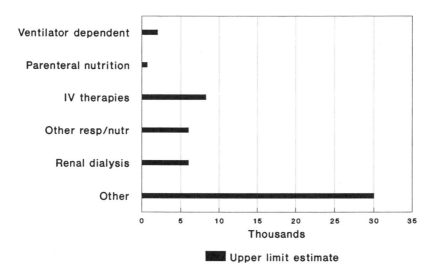

Figure 1-2. Numbers of children dependent on technology, United States, 1987 (U.S. Congress, 1987).

The Rights of Families

Sensitivity to the rights of people coping with disadvantage has developed over the past three decades. Increased attention and services for mentally ill and retarded people, which developed during the Kennedy Administration; landmark civil rights legislation in the mid-1960s; and expanded research in child psychology and education are among the events leading to Public Law 94–142, the Education of the Handicapped Act of 1975 (Martin, no date; Rieser, 1986). Other efforts at community, state, and federal levels, such as the extension and implementation of Section 504 of the Rehabilitation Act, have also increased the national emphasis on the rights of handicapped individuals and their families. Health care generally has been marked by growing consumerism and greater participation of families and patients in their own health care. Thus, a growing number of families with hospitalized children who have complex medical problems have demanded the opportunity to treat their children at home to foster more appropriate growth and development (Association for the Care of Children's Health, 1984; Stein, 1987). Family advocacy programs, such as the Technical Assistance to Parents Program, the Federation for Children with Special Needs in Boston, the SKIP (Sick Kids need Involved Persons) program with its several local chapters, and Pilot Parents' groups, have supported greater awareness of family rights through parent training, advocacy programs, self-help groups, and programs that encourage active collaboration between health professionals and parents. All of these activities express a belief that children's growth and development is best nurtured in their own homes and communities rather than in hospitals or institutions.

The Growth of Technology

Technological advances have also stimulated growth in home care for children with severe illnesses. Generally, these technological advances greatly improve the lives of these children and their families. Youngsters with severe long-term illnesses face markedly lower mortality rates than they did 20 years ago. Today, although some chronically ill children die from their illness, at least 80 percent survive to young adulthood (Gortmaker, 1985; Gortmaker & Sappenfield, 1984). Significant handicap or disability often accompanies survival, and some children with long-term illnesses require in-home health services of varying complexity.

Technology has become increasingly portable, and its use no longer needs to be restricted to the hospital. Many antibiotics that must be given intravenously can be administered at home with special equipment (Stiver et al.,

1982). Youngsters with hemophilia, who previously had to receive replacement blood factors in hospitals for their bleeding episodes, can now administer blood products at home themselves (Smith & Levine, 1984). Children requiring long-term complex nutritional support by IV line now receive these services at home (Robinovitch, 1981). Large hospital-based ventilators have been replaced with smaller portable models that allow children who are ventilator-dependent to be cared for at home, school, or even the shopping mall (Burr et al., 1983; Donn, 1982; Kacmarek & Thompson, 1986). These examples illustrate some of the new technologies that permit the expansion of home care.

With these new technologies and parental involvement in children's health care has come greater professional comfort with out-of-hospital care. In the past, physicians assumed that complex care always had to take place in a hospital. Now they willingly explore alternative sites, both outpatient and home- and community-based, for these services (Edwardson, 1985).

Technological advances, however, do not always benefit families. There is evidence of a "technological imperative" that at times drives services in ways that may be counter to the best functioning of families. The emphasis on technology often outweighs efforts to help families cope with their technology-dependent children. Newborn intensive care units, for example, commonly focus on maintaining an infant's respiratory status or hemodynamic balance and neglect supporting families and teaching them ways of caring for their child. Further, newborn programs place little emphasis on follow-up, such as planning for comprehensive, community-based services after discharge and monitoring the infant's progress in light of the special risks children face after leaving the intensive care unit (Bauchner, Brown, & Peskin, 1988; Hoffman & Bennett, 1990; Ludman, Lansdown, & Spitz, 1989). Many of the gains from the use of complex technology in the child's first months of life may be reduced or eliminated by lack of basic follow-up services, care that tends to get short shrift in the context of high-tech treatment. Similarly, home-based services may depend on the availability of complex equipment in the home, without first assuring that the machinery works over time and that the people in the home are competent and comfortable using the equipment.

The technological imperative goes beyond the relative emphasis of high technology over low technology. In many cases, major technologies are used in the home when their use may not be in the best interest of the child. Just as the issue of when to use or not use technological methods in hospitals to save lives creates complicated ethical questions, so too there may be a drive to apply home- and community-based technologies without fully weighing the consequences and the implications for the child and the family. New technologies *have* led to great improvement in many lives; yet for many families, indiscriminate use of new technologies creates burdens that they and their children are unable to handle.

Policies and programs have failed to keep pace with these technological advances. Furthermore, families often lack access to an adequately broad range of services, and the shift to home care may increase both out-of-pocket expenses and opportunity costs for families. The emphasis on high technology also leaves many other equally important services unsupported. And for many children, access to technologies may be curtailed when they grow older. The great improvements in survival rates mean that many youngsters ''age out'' of programs when they become adolescents and young adults. They lose benefits under their parents' health insurance but continue to have major health needs. Public support through maternal and child health programs may have age cutoffs; rehabilitation and family income support programs may wither because in years past the expectation was that these young people would not survive and need these programs.

Cost Containment

The third impetus behind the growth of home care for chronically ill children has been cost containment. Rapidly escalating costs of health care have made cost containment and the search for the lowest-cost alternative the central driving force in American health policy over the past decade (Enthoven & Kronick, 1989). The 2 to 4 percent of children with severe long-term illnesses use a disproportionate percentage of pediatric health services, conservatively at least ten times the per capita utilization of children without apparent illnesses (Butler et al., 1985a).

Hospitalization accounts for roughly one-half of all child health expenditures, and again severely ill children utilize a relatively high percentage of all childhood hospitalizations. Decreasing the likelihood of hospitalization would be expected to produce sizable cost savings. The 1982 Surgeon General's workshop on children with handicaps and their families took as its main model the problem of respirator-dependent children (U.S. Department of Health and Human Services, 1982). Hospital care for each of these children costs roughly $200,000 or more per year. Data presented at the workshop suggested that providing high-quality, home-based services is much cheaper, on the order of $80,000 per year. In this and other cases, the cost-saving potential of home care has become increasingly attractive to private and governmental payers and to cost-conscious employers.

DEFINITIONS

The children who are the focus of this book require special medical, nursing, or other health care services at home in order to grow and prosper. These youngsters fall into two groups covering a wide variety of conditions. Children in the first group are technology dependent, relying on mechanical supports to replace or supplement the function of their own organs. These children include, for example, those who are ventilator dependent; those requiring special support for nutrition, through the use of either a gastrostomy, a surgically prepared opening through the abdomen directly into the stomach, to facilitate feeding, or IV feedings (parenteral nutrition); or children who have tracheostomies, openings directly into the trachea (windpipe) to facilitate breathing. This list of technologies is not exhaustive but illustrates the needs of some of these children. The second group of children in this study are those whose medical conditions, while not necessarily requiring the support of medical technologies, place major responsibility for ongoing care and treatment on families. Examples of youngsters in this latter group are those with cystic fibrosis who require frequent chest physiotherapy, children with spina bifida who require intermittent catheterization to empty their bladders, and children with cancer who need extensive treatment and long-term monitoring of their conditions.

Other terms require definition as they are used in this text: care at home, severe illness, families, community-based services, and case management and care coordination.

We define *home care* as services and procedures that help the family function effectively in meeting the varied needs of an ill child at home and in the community. The therapeutic goals for chronically ill children and their families include integration into community life, enhancing child and family responsibility for self-care, and optimal social and educational development. This definition includes the provision of technological services and direct health care in the home, but it extends much further. Direct services—including nursing care (changing dressings, administering medicines, educating family members around care issues), physical therapy, and developmental services—are part of the package of home care. Yet the range of services also includes those that enhance the family's strengths and develop a nurturing home environment. Others define home care more narrowly as specific health services provided in the home. As used in this text, the term refers to the broader definition described above.

By *severe illness* we mean a health condition that interferes on a regular daily basis with the activities in which children normally participate; one that creates need for attention from a variety of health and related providers; that requires extensive, long-term, or multiple hospitalizations; or that requires recurrent or continuous in-home health services. We use the adjectives "severe," "chronic," and "long-term" and the nouns "illness" and "health condition" interchangeably in this book.

By *families* we mean the constellation of people living together for mutual support and caretaking. This definition recognizes that many children live with both biological parents and many do not, and it encompasses such arrangements as children living in foster care or with their extended families.

By *community-based services* we mean services and procedures provided outside the hospital or other institutions. Community-based services include those related to a child's special needs and other community services (schools, recreation, etc.) available to all families. Although many technological services are specific to the idiosyncracies of individual conditions, many needed services are generic, and it is these especially that can be provided at the community level.

The terms *case management* and *care coordination*, which are used here synonymously, have almost as many definitions as there are clients receiving the service and providers for it. Gittler and Colton's review (1986) provides several examples. The Florida Title V program, the Children's Medical Service, defines case management as the "means of achieving service integration through the linkage of the service systems with a consumer and coordination of various components to achieve a successful outcome." The definition further explains case management as "the process of planning and assuring comprehensive health care services for [CMS] patients for the purpose . . . of achieving maximum individual potential" (p. 10). The Division of Services for Crippled Children of Michigan views case management "as a process by which families are assisted to gain skills and independence in problem solving, management of the human service system and self-advocacy" (p. 90).

Our definition of case management or care coordination encompasses all of these concepts: linking families with services, coordinating services, maximizing a child's growth and development through the provision of appropriate services, helping and educating families, and monitoring the outcomes for both children and families. Of special importance is the education of families: information about the child's conditions, how best to care for the child, how to manage the service systems to obtain appropriate care, and how to carry out the responsibilities of case management independent of a professional service provider. This concept of case management or care coordination is distinct from the "case management" service provided by many insurers, which restricts access to care to reduce costs. Such case management is more appropriately termed "benefits management" and does not meet the definition of case management or care coordination used in this book.

LONG-TERM CARE FOR THE ELDERLY: IS IT THE SAME OR DIFFERENT FOR CHILDREN?

Just as more children survive with complex medical conditions and require long-term health care, the number of elderly Americans who need long-term care has risen and will increase markedly over the next several decades (Manton, 1989). Elderly people and severely ill children have many similar long-term care needs. Both groups depend on technologies and on caretaking from other people. Both require a broad scope of services, including attention not only to health and medical needs but also to social and psychological issues related to long-term care. Yet there are important ways in which they differ.

First, long-term care for the elderly has a primary base of financial support in Medicare. This federal health insurance program leaves virtually no elderly person uninsured and provides an important economic base on which to build comprehensive long-term care financing (General Accounting Office, 1986; Koren, 1986). This is not to say that Medicare benefits, especially for long-term care, are adequate to meet the needs of many of our nation's elderly. Rather, it is to stress that no similar insurance program exists for children. Many youngsters lack basic insurance to pay for fundamental health services, much less the more complex care required by their severe chronic illnesses (McManus, 1989; Rosenbaum, 1988).

Second, the goals of home care for the elderly differ from those for children with severe illnesses. Although for many elderly, home care may have a rehabilitative focus, for most the goal of home care is to diminish the need for institutional or hospital services, or at least to postpone the time when institutional services may be needed (Branch et al., 1988; Mor, Wachtel, & Kidder, 1985). Although many home-care services for children are provided in the context of reducing hospitalization, the major goals of home care for children fit into a scenario of habilitation, with the focus on integrating children into the community and encouraging their development so that they may become full participating members of society.

Third, society has different perceptions of who should bear responsibility for care of the elderly and for care of the young. Society's assumption of responsibility for medical care for the elderly is followed by a growing consensus concerning social responsibility for ensuring some level of long-term care for the elderly. The elderly often have an aged family: The spouse may be deceased and the children, on whom responsibility for care would otherwise fall, are middle-aged or elderly themselves and are unable or unwilling to care for an ailing parent. Thus, the social commitment reflects in part the belief that many elderly citizens lack family members to provide supportive long-term care. Society assumes no similar responsibility for the medical care of children or for their long-term treatment. The prevailing assumption is that the child with a complex medical condition has an intact family with a mother at home who is able to meet her youngster's needs. This assumption ignores the realities of today's family structure (e.g., single and divorced parents), the increased reliance on two incomes with the mother working outside the home to make ends meet, and the enormously complex technical requirements of long-term care for a child with a chronic health condition. Children with long-term illness live outside the framework of public awareness, even though youngsters like Jack and Philip (described earlier) illustrate compelling needs that are best achieved through a societal commitment to help their families meet their responsibilities. As a nation, we have begun to accept social responsibility for the care of the elderly through Medicare and national long-term care initiatives. As a nation, we expect all families, regardless of their need or ability, to care for their children with little public support.

Finally, major developmental issues frame the organization and delivery of home-care services for children in a way different from issues for the elderly. A child's care occurs in the context of a rapidly growing and developing person. Although chronic illness may impede their progress, most children face the same opportunities as other youngsters for development and productive lives over many decades. The elderly, nearing the end of their lives, have different developmental needs. By necessity, developmental needs greatly influence the provision of home-care services for children. Attention to developmental issues, through assessment, planning, and education, will help the child achieve his or her best possible functioning.

THE STUDY

Home- and community-based care for children with complex illnesses gained increasing public attention during the 1980s. Evaluation of the Pediatric Home Care Program at Albert Einstein College of Medicine (New York City) provided the first careful, in-depth analysis of the ways in which home care may work for children and families (Stein & Jessop, 1984). The Vanderbilt University (Nashville, Tenn.) study of public policies affecting chronically ill children and their families, sponsored by the U.S. Department of Health and Human Services and the Department of Education, provided an overview of programmatic and policy recommendations to improve the lives of both the increasing numbers of children who survive with severe long-term illnesses and their families (Hobbs, Perrin, & Ireys, 1985). The Bureau of Maternal and

Child Health of the U.S. Department of Health and Human Services broadened community, policymaker, provider, and consumer awareness through a series of regional, local, and national conferences in 1984 and 1985 regarding varied aspects of the lives of children with severe long-term health conditions. During the early 1980s, Surgeon General C. Everett Koop sponsored three national workshops on technology-dependent children and on children with severe health impairments. Federal action on catastrophic health insurance for the elderly in 1986 stimulated interest in children's catastrophic health conditions. Congressional inquiry into the adequacy of home care for the chronically ill young followed in 1987 and resulted in the introduction of legislation to improve access to home care (Senate bill 87–1537). In 1987, Health and Human Services Secretary Otis R. Bowen established the Task Force on Technology-Dependent Children, which promulgated recommendations for federal policy (U.S. Department of Health and Human Services, 1988). Recent changes in the maternal and child health block grant require that state agencies provide leadership in developing systems of care for these children, including more appropriate home- and community-based services.

These activities have clarified the nature of the barriers to optimal care of these children and their families. Key failings have been the lack of standards, policies, and financial support for the provision of out-of-hospital, home-, and community-based services for these children. As more of the children survive into adulthood, more of their care should be provided in less intensive settings, and the main goal should be the integration of the children and their families into all regular aspects of community life. We undertook this study of policies regarding home care for children to bring the opportunities for improved family life to a wider and more influential audience.

Examination of policies and programs for home care for children with severe illnesses, on which this book is based, was carried out over three years, from mid-1985 through mid-1988. The study had three components. First, we explored in depth the knowledge base concerning home care for children. This literature review examined descriptive and research studies of programs for youngsters. Second, we asked experts in medicine, nursing, family advocacy, social services, and health policy to identify exemplary programs across the nation that provided high-quality home-care services for severely ill children and their families. We reviewed program descriptions, annual reports, and, in the rare instances where they were available, program evaluations so as to identify key programmatic features and policy options. Third, we used our reviews of the literature and programs as the basis for selecting ten home-care programs at which we conducted site visits to gain firsthand knowledge about policy and programmatic issues. The literature review and site visits are described in greater detail below.

Literature Review

A review of the literature demonstrated that little has been systematically and substantially studied in this important realm. Much of what has been described is anecdotal; little is supported by serious analysis or careful research. The paucity of the literature partly reflects the fact that interest in home care for children with complex medical conditions is of relatively recent vintage. Literature on the effects of severe chronic childhood illness on families and children is sparse (see Burr, 1985; Hobbs, Perrin, & Ireys, 1985; Stein, 1989). Even fewer articles report the experiences of families in caring for these children at home and in their communities (Hochstadt & Yost, 1991).

A few reports examine home care for children with specific illnesses, such as hemophilia (Kaufert, 1980; LeQuesne et al., 1974; McKenzie, Fie, & Van Eys, 1974; Smith & Levine, 1984; Strawczynski et al., 1973); cystic fibrosis (Oppenheimer & Rucker, 1980); and cancer (Strayer, Kisker, & Fethke, 1980), particularly in the terminal stage (Edwardson, 1983, 1985; Fergusson & Hobbie, 1985; Lauer et al., 1983; Moldow & Martinson, 1980; Moldow et al., 1982). Other reports discuss specific procedures for children at home, for example, tracheostomies (Foster & Hoskins, 1981; Newton et al., 1982; Ruben et al., 1982); hemodialysis (Blagg et al., 1970; Delano et al., 1981); peritoneal dialysis (Counts et al., 1973; Goldberg, Baugham, & Wombolt, 1980); parenteral nutrition (Robinovitch, 1981); and intravenous antibiotics (Rucker & Harrison, 1974; Stiver et al., 1982).

Descriptions of programs that support families who are providing care at home for children with a variety of severe chronic health conditions comprise a small body of literature (Adam, 1989; Bock, 1983; Case & Matthews, 1983; Freedman & Pierce, 1989; Pierce & Freedman, 1983; Stein & Jessop, 1984). The Surgeon General's Workshop (U.S. Department of Health and Human Services, 1982) focused attention on children dependent on various technologies, particularly respirators and ventilators. Home care for technology-assisted children has been the subject of reports in the mid-1980s (Burr et al., 1983; Feinberg, 1985; Goldberg et al., 1984; Thorp, 1987; U.S. Congress, 1987) and of three demonstration programs funded by the Office of Maternal and Child Health of the U.S. Department of Health and Human Services (with the agency's discretionary funds for Special Programs of Regional and National Significance, SPRANS) and evaluated by the Center for Health Administration Studies at the University of Chicago (Aday, Aitken, & Wegener, 1988). Among the few research studies are the randomized control trial of the Pediatric Home Care Program (Stein & Jessop, 1984), the University of Chicago's rigorous evaluation of the SPRANS-funded demonstration programs, and a systematic study of mothers of ventilator-dependent children

(Thorp, 1987). In sum, the literature, although rich in anecdotal reports, contains little empirical evidence of the effects on families of caring at home for children with long-term illnesses.

Site Visits

Of the over one hundred home-care programs nominated by experts as exemplary, ten were selected for in-depth study. To capture the experience of a broad variety of program models, we considered a number of distinguishing features in choosing the sites. The factors were: (1) population served, including whether the program served children with only one health condition or chronically ill children defined generically; (2) organizational locus, that is, whether the program was hospital-based, free-standing, or part of another system such as a prepaid health care plan; (3) organizational structure, that is, whether the program was governmental, private not-for-profit, or private for-profit; (4) services offered, that is, whether programs were procedure-specific or comprehensive, and whether they emphasized case management or direct services; (5) approach to service delivery, that is, by individuals or teams; and (6) geographic location, namely region of the country and whether the area served was urban or rural. Programs selected for review represent diversity on each factor.

Visits to each site were conducted by two of the authors during 1986 and 1987. Visits were designed to enrich our understanding about elements of best practice and about obstacles to successful home care. Each visit was preceded by extensive preparation to help the authors understand the organizational, service, and financial issues facing the program. During the site visits, we met with families, children, program staff, referral providers including physicians, schools, early intervention personnel, and funding agencies.

Prior to the site visits, we developed and field-tested a series of interview schedules for each of these groups of respondents. These interview schedules guided the interviews and facilitated the collection of comparable information from diverse programs. Because many questions were deliberately open-ended, a great deal of rich material emerged in areas that the questionnaires did not anticipate. The families whom we interviewed are not a scientifically valid sample of families with children in home care. Rather, they were selected by program personnel because they were judged to be roughly representative of families who have succeeded in meeting the challenges of home care and were able to convey their experiences to us. Most families had at least some form of public or private health insurance for their child; many were poor; and generally these families *did* receive services and some coordination of their care. The location of the family meeting and the independence of the interview from program staff varied by site. Some families were visited at their homes but others were interviewed at the programs' offices, mainly when scheduled appointments coincided with our visit. Similarly, some families were interviewed in the presence of program staff while others were interviewed privately by the investigators. The inherent biases in family selection and the interviewing process are recognized but were outside our control. Nevertheless, we believe that the family interviews provided an accurate portrayal of their experiences.

The site visits provided a body of compelling information. We found an ecological niche of a complex nature, one in which children with severe illnesses received attention to their developmental, health care, social, and psychological needs, usually in the context of interventions that strengthened the families' abilities to care for their children and to nurture their growth. Professionals and families in the ten home-care programs shared their experiences with us with extraordinary generosity and shaped our understanding of the issues in providing home care for children with chronic health conditions and their families. A brief description of each program follows.

Children's Memorial Hospital in Chicago provides services, including discharge planning, to children with severe chronic illnesses. Patients include a large number of ventilator-dependent children, many of whom would be eligible for the Illinois Division of Services to Crippled Children's home-care program, which is described below. Our site visit concentrated on the discharge planning program for ventilator-dependent children, which has the objective of preparing families for their child's safe discharge from hospital to home. To achieve this objective, the hospital has a clear, comprehensive plan of action that spells out time frames and delegation of responsibility. It uses a step-down unit to help parents and children make the transition from hospital to home. In this unit, children have more freedom to explore and are prepared for the differences between life in the hospital and life at home. The planning process, which trains parents to take over the care of their children, emphasizes management of physical care and technology.

Coordinating Center for Home and Community Care, Inc., provides care coordination and monitoring for children in the state of Maryland who are dependent on a variety of technologies, including respirators. An independent, free-standing corporation, the Coordinating Center is a consortium of five academic medical centers, state Medicaid and Crippled Children's Services agencies, and private health insurers. Funded initially by a federal SPRANS grant, the center now receives reimbursement for 41 of the 61 children enrolled through a Medicaid waiver and for the rest from private insurance companies. The focus of the center's program is case management, with the goal of enabling parents to take charge of their child's care. Center staff includes nurse coordinators, family resource and educational coordinators, a medical director, policy analyst, and financial coordinator.

Coordination for Pediatrics (*COPE*) *at New York Hospital* is one of four demonstration projects of the Coordination of Care for Chronically Ill Children Program established in the mid-1980s with funding from the New York State Department of Health. COPE is staffed with a full-time nurse and a part-time pediatrician and psychological/educational specialist. The caseload, about 90 low-income families, includes children with a variety of chronic health conditions. The principal service provided to families is coordination of the care delivered by New York Hospital medical and surgical services and facilitation of access to community resources, with emphasis on empowerment of parents to take charge of their youngster's care.

The *Illinois Division of Services to Crippled Children* (*DSCC*) *program for ventilator-dependent children* is one of three demonstration programs for this group of youngsters funded by the Bureau of Maternal and Child Health of the U.S. Department of Health and Human Services. The goal of the demonstration programs is to gain experience in supporting families in caring for ventilator-dependent children at home rather than in the hospital. At the time of our study, the Illinois program was in the planning stages. A major thrust of the program was to assure that home-care services would receive reimbursement from the state's Medicaid program and other third-party payers by the establishment of innovative, cooperative interagency agreements. When in full operation, the agency planned to provide case management as the major service for families of ventilator-dependent children throughout the state. Subsequent to the site visit in September 1986, the program achieved its operational goals (Bilotti, 1989).

Iowa Child Health Specialty Clinics is the Title V Program for Children with Special Health Care Needs for the state of Iowa. Based at the state university in Iowa City, it operates the Home Care Monitoring Program (HCMP) and Home Care Support Program (HCSP) in the context of a network of regional centers and mobile clinics that serve children with a broad range of medical, developmental, behavioral, and educational problems. HCMP, centrally based in Iowa City, provides case coordination for medically complex children and their families. The staff of two nurses and a parent advocate work within the university hospital to facilitate discharge of children with complex medical needs and to coordinate with the child's community in developing a service plan for care at home. HCSP nurses in the regional centers provide ongoing case coordination and family support. Medicaid funds (through a waiver for home- and community-based care or eligibility for Supplemental Security Income [SSI]), reimbursement from private insurance plans, and patient fees pay for the services for approximately a hundred children and their families.

La Rabida Hospital is a 77-bed chronic-care hospital for children that is affiliated with the Department of Pediatrics at the University of Chicago. A central element of La Rabida's services is its comprehensive discharge planning program, which prepares families to care for their medically complex, often technology-dependent children at home. The discharge planning process begins as soon as possible after the child is admitted and preferably before the child is transferred to La Rabida from the acute-care hospital. A team composed of a physician, nurse, social worker, and rehabilitation specialist works with the family to design the plan and train the parents to care for the child at home. Coordination with community health care providers, schools, and other services is provided by La Rabida clinical nurse specialists, who often serve as case managers.

The *Pediatric Home Care Program at the Albert Einstein College of Medicine* provides a comprehensive range of services including primary care, home visits, counseling, care management, advocacy, liaison with schools and other community resources, and, most important, family education (Adam, 1989). The program serves about 90 low-income, chronically ill children and their families who live in the borough of the Bronx, in New York City. Families with multiple problems and dysfunctions are given priority for admission to the Pediatric Home Care Program. The staff includes primary care pediatricians, pediatric nurse practitioners, a social worker, and a consulting child psychiatrist. Each family's care is delivered by a multidisciplinary team led by a pediatric nurse practitioner. The major payer for almost all families at this facility is Medicaid.

The *Regional Comprehensive Hemophilia Diagnostic and Treatment Center at New York Hospital–Cornell Medical Center* serves 287 patients with hemophilia and related diseases from the greater New York area. The program provides access to a wide range of providers in a single, several-hour visit. Services include genetic counseling, hematology, orthopedics, oral surgery, dental hygiene, nursing, social work, physical therapy, and vocational counseling. Policies of third-party payers, which include private health insurance plans and Medicaid, preclude the provision of psychosocial services. The center has been a leader in bringing the technological breakthrough of home administration of blood products to patients and their families.

Rural Efforts to Assist Children at Home (REACH), a project of the Florida Children's Medical Services, was begun as a demonstration program that organized a broad range of services to families who care for complex, chronically ill children in rural north Florida (Freedman & Pierce, 1989). Subsequently, the program has been implemented statewide. Services, which emphasize case management and empowerment of families to care for their children, are provided by nurses who live in the local communities and who are trained and supervised by REACH staff located in Gainesville. Family disintegration, chaotic home life, and severity of the child's illness are factors that are taken into account in admission to REACH. All families are low-income and financially eligible for Children's Medical Services.

The *Visiting Nurse Service (VNS) of New York* serves the boroughs of Queens, Manhattan, and the Bronx. VNS has a separately identifiable Maternal and Child Health–Pediatrics Division. The children served by the program have multiple chronic illnesses and live in poor or near-poor families. In 1985, the Pediatric Program provided 28,000 home visits by registered nurses, physical and occupational therapists, speech therapists, social workers, and home health aides and was projected to grow substantially over the years. The services, which include physical assessments of the children, monitoring, and direct care, are procedure-oriented. Services provided are those reimbursed by the VNS's principal payers, Medicaid and private health insurance, and do not include care coordination and psychosocial services.

We have shortened or abbreviated the names of the programs when we cite them in the text (Table 1–2). Characteristics of the programs selected for the study are listed in Table 1–3.

Table 1-2. Programs Surveyed at 10 Study Sites

Programs	Shortened or abbreviated name
Children's Memorial Hospital, Chicago	Chicago Children's
Coordinating Center for Home and Community Care, Inc., Maryland	Maryland
Coordination for Pediatrics, New York Hospital	COPE
Illinois Division of Services to Crippled Children	Illinois
Iowa Child Health Specialty Clinics	Iowa
La Rabida Hospital	La Rabida
Pediatric Home Care, Albert Einstein College of Medicine	Einstein
Regional Comprehensive Hemophilia Diagnostic and Treatment Center, New York Hospital–Cornell Medical Center	Hemophilia Center
Rural Efforts to Assist Children at Home	REACH
Visiting Nurse Service of New York	VNS

Table 1-3. Characteristics of Programs in the Study

Program Characteristics	Chicago Children's	Maryland	COPE	Illinois	Iowa	La Rabida	Einstein	Hemophilia Center	REACH	VNS
CHARACTERISTICS OF THE POPULATION SERVED										
health condition specific	X							X		
all chronic illnesses		X	X	X	X	X	X		X	X
ORGANIZATIONAL LOCUS										
hospital-based	X	X	X			X	X	X		
free-standing										
part of larger system				X	X				X	X
ORGANIZATIONAL STRUCTURE										
governmental				X	X					
private nonprofit	X	X	X			X	X	X	X	X
SERVICES OFFERED										
procedure-specific										
comprehensive	X	X	X	X	X	X	X	X	X	X
METHOD OF SERVICE DELIVERY										
case management		X	X	X	X	X	X	X	X	X
direct services	X		X		X	X	X	X	X	X
SERVICE DELIVERY APPROACH										
individual providers			X							
teams	X	X		X	X	X	X	X	X	X
REGION SERVED										
urban	X	X	X	X	X	X	X	X		X
rural	X	X	X	X	X				X	

Evidence from the Study

The consistency with which the experiences and problems of families were recounted in both the literature and the site visits is impressive. Although both sources have important limitations, the site visits strongly confirm the written reports. Similar issues were raised by families and children who represent a broad range of health conditions; who live in communities that run the gamut from relatively resource-rich suburbs to poverty-stricken rural areas to deteriorated and destabilized inner cities; whose economic circumstances and family structures are diverse; and whose offspring children have been in care at home for varying lengths of time. Observations by professionals about the experiences of families were also similar, regardless of the particular site or discipline. The repetition of themes, with variations, in the literature and by families and professionals in home-care programs across the nation lends validity to our analyses of issues in the care of severely health-impaired children at home. We quote extensively from these visits in the chapters that follow and indicate the source of each quote. To protect the privacy of both families and children, we have changed their names and altered their stories when we describe or quote them in this text; however, the underlying issues remain intact.

The literature and our visits with families and program personnel persuade us that enough is known to define key issues and to make firm and positive proposals to meet the needs of children with severe illnesses and their families. Further investigation is clearly needed to understand what works and for which families, but the lack of research should not prevent the nation from creating appropriate, cost-effective, humane, compassionate responses to the needs of families.

2

The Impact on Families

Sally Gannon was well until 7 months of age, when she suffered a severe injury in which her neck was caught between the crib slats, causing the loss of oxygen to her brain for an extended period of time. Sally was in an intensive care unit (ICU) for three weeks and then in a rehabilitation unit for five additional months. Initially, Sally's family found it difficult to cope with the change in their daughter's situation and with the unpredictability of her eventual developmental status.

Now 4 years old, Sally has made little developmental progress since the accident, although she is just learning to vocalize. Her occasional seizures are well controlled with medicines. She has a tracheostomy that requires suctioning. When she gets a viral cold or similar infection, fluid and mucus clog her breathing tract and she requires extensive nursing care. Except when her seizures act up or she has bad respiratory problems, her condition is fairly stable. She is unable to control her body functions, and she must be helped with all feeding.

Sally's parents both work outside the home. Their extensive and effective home-care program provides 16 to 20 hours per day of in-home nursing care for Sally. Sally's room is on the main floor of the house, and the closet holds all of her necessary feeding and lung-care items. Her parents' room is on the floor below, separate from the activity surrounding Sally's continuing care. Mr. and Mrs. Gannon thus have privacy, while maintaining an active role in Sally's care. In the early days after their daughter's injury, the Gannon family experienced marital strain, arguing about how to resolve problems about their home life and Sally's care at home. Over the past two years, they have been very happy with the arrangement that allows them to continue their lives outside the home while providing a good deal of nurturing care to their daughter. Last summer, Sally's parents and her 13-year-old sister, Jean, were able to take a two-week vacation by arranging for Sally's grandparents to stay at the house with continuing nursing services.

Jean participates in many aspects of family life, including providing some care to Sally. Jean loves her sister and is proud of Sally's recent successes in vocalization. Jean carries on an active school life, generally getting As and Bs in class, and has recently become interested in dating boys for which her parents feel she is too young. She is an energetic and interesting girl, having grown well under the guidance of her family.

Now that she is embarking on adolescence, Jean has been experiencing more problems dealing with her feelings about having an impaired sister. Jean resents the extra attention that Sally gets and feels that she is being neglected and overprotected by her parents. Her homeroom teacher recently noticed disturbing changes in Jean's school performance and immediately spoke with the Gannons about his concerns. As a result, Jean is receiving counseling and seems to be coming to terms with her new ambivalence about her family situation.

The Gannon family has done well caring for Sally because of their strengths and the availability of good support services. Their program is broad enough that Jean's special needs at the time of transition to adolescence also receive attention. The goal of policies and programs should be to maximize the strengths and abilities of families like Sally's to care for and nurture their children. Formulation of effective home-care policies and programs requires an understanding of the effects on family life of providing care at home for children with long-term, severe health conditions. Stated most simply, "The key players are the family" (Kacmarek & Thompson, 1986, p. 605). We describe here the experiences of families, focusing especially on the issues they encounter in home care.

PARENTS' PREFERENCES

Most families whose children have severe, complex medical conditions believe that having their children with them at home rather than in the hospital is better for themselves and their children. One mother interviewed expressed her feelings succinctly: "Home care is a life saver" (Hemophilia Center). At the same time, the home care of children with serious, long-term health conditions strains family functioning.

Several studies of parents whose children require respiratory support have noted families' contradictory feelings about home care. A study of Massachusetts families with ventilator-dependent children concluded thus:

Without exception, the parents expressed their belief that bringing their children home from the hospital has had a beneficial effect on family relations. All have commented on the strain of long-term daily hospital visits and the difficulty they have imposed on their other children. . . . The positive feelings of the parents should not be construed as suggesting that they are unaware of the effects of this unusual situation on their own lives. (Burr et al., 1983, p. 1321)

Aday and colleagues (1988), who interviewed the parents of 132 ventilator-assisted children, noted:

Caregivers think it is better for the children to be at home, though it often makes it hard on the family. The vast majority of families agreed that their children did much better in terms of their overall physical, intellectual, and emotional development and well-being at home and they "felt more like a family" compared to when the child was in the hospital. These perceptions were, however, tempered by the day-to-day stress VAC's [ventilator-assisted children's] families and principal caregivers also reported in having the children at home. (p. 326).

Other researchers echo these findings. "While home care may have . . . psycho-social benefits for children, it is not without great cost to the family" (Thorp, 1987, p. 48). Families mainly prefer home care because of the benefits they perceive for their children's development and their own well-being (Anderson, 1985; Lauer et al., 1983; Oster, 1985; Strawczynski et al., 1973) even though the stresses are great.

Stein (1987) observed:

Policy must recognize that the burdens of a child's medical condition and its technical as well as emotional characteristics place a great deal of extra stress on the family unit. This factor is the one most often ignored in discussions of home care policy. Regardless of the specific medical diagnoses and the technical, medical, and nursing tasks that are necessary for the care of the child, the presence of serious ongoing illness creates extra burdens. (p. 26)

Care at home may extend the length of life of some children who would otherwise die more quickly in a hospital or other institution. Clinicians and families have observed that when children move from hospital to home, their conditions often improve in the stimulating, nurturing home environment. Yet parental expectations and decisions may be based on information on survival from hospital settings. The benefits and stresses may therefore last longer than the family expected. An important element in planning for home care, then, is the provision of realistic estimates to parents concerning the effect of home care on their child's prognosis.

Although home care offers potential benefits for family life and children's development, some families may be unable to handle home care of a severely ill child. Families who live in deep poverty in the inner cities face immense obstacles to providing adequate care. As middle-class families moved from urban ghettoes to more prosperous neighborhoods, they left behind increased rates of teenage pregnancy, female-headed households, drug abuse, and welfare dependency and declining basic institutions—churches, schools, health, and recreational facilities (Gorham & Glazer, 1976; McGeary & Lynn, 1988; Wilson, 1987). Few resources are in place that can be marshalled to enable families to manage their children's complex health conditions.

The higher incidence of chronic health conditions among poor children, many of whom are concentrated in communities with destabilized social institutions, challenges even the most heroic families and home care programs (Stein & Jessop, 1985). The situation is bleak for the disproportionate number of very young, poor mothers with premature babies and for those whose infants are affected by maternal use of alcohol and drugs (Brody, 1991). "Not all homes are appropriate for the adequate management of chronic illness. Some home situations can be improved with appropriate support services. However, some children must remain in institutions for years, for social, educational, or developmental reasons" (Goldberg et al., 1984, p. 793). The difficulties that families may face should not by themselves require long-term hospitalization for their children. Group homes or foster care settings usually offer better alternatives for the care and growth of these youngsters.

Families across the socioeconomic spectrum are engaged in home care. "With the exception of medical stabilization, the capability of the family to care for the [ventilator-dependent] child is by far the most critical factor [in successful home care]. An enthusiastic and supportive family, capable of learning and participating actively in the care of the child, is essential" (Kacmarek & Thompson, 1986, p. 610). The relationship between socioeconomic status and the ability to manage home care is poorly understood. Studies of the question have contradictory results. Some have found that middle-class families with relatively good resources are more capable of caring for severely ill children at home than are single-parent or lower-income families.

Frates and colleagues (1985) describe 54 children on home ventilation. Ninety percent were from middle- or upper-income families, and 80 percent were from two-parent families. Similarly, Kacmarek and Thompson (1986, p. 610), state, "It appears that most families who are capable and willing to care for this type of child are from middle or upper social class socioeconomic levels and are two parent households." In contrast, Feinberg (1985) observes:

Contrary to conventional wisdom, middle and upper class families often have greater difficulty contending with the ongoing impact of the medically fragile child than lower middle class families. The former category is used to maintaining control over their lives, resuming careers, and enjoying varying degrees of self-indulgence. Families that have fewer options and have lower expectations of self-actualization are better prepared to cope with the unpredictability of the medically fragile child. (p. 41)

The fairly large number of poor families involved can be attributed in part to the fact that many home care programs are financed by Medicaid, which limits the income and other financial resources that families may have in order to qualify for services. The families we interviewed represented disparate socio-economic conditions. They were middle-class families in a suburban Iowa subdivision, a poverty-stricken family living in a house trailer in rural Florida, blue-collar families in Queens, New York, duplexes, and families just getting by on public assistance in a housing project in the Bronx (New York). How well families manage home care appears to be related less to their affluence per se than to a combination of other factors.

Some of these factors were identified by Stein and Jessop (1984) at the Einstein Pediatric Home Care program. These researchers have conducted the most extensive empirical research on children's home care to date. They examined how the child's health condition and the family's resources and coping ability affected the ability to provide successful home care. The measures examined concerning the child's health condition were need for medical and nursing care; physical and developmental deficits; level of functioning; disruptions in the family's daily routines that home care entails; and the psychological burden of the child's prognosis. The assessment of families' coping abilities included the primary caretaker's (usually the mother's) physical, emotional, and educational resources; the social supports and help available; and competing demands for the family's time and energy. As Stein (1985) concluded:

A successful home care experience for a child depends on careful assessment of both sets of factors and on a balance between the resources and the burden. The role of home care is to help equalize the relationship between the burden and the family's resources. While all families whose children have a high burden may need some type of home care program in order to consider managing their chronically ill child at home, those with lowest resources and highest burden may not be able to do so, even with a strong program, and those with a less burdensome condition and somewhat greater resources may be able to manage with a less supportive program. (p. 92)

EFFECTS ON FAMILIES

Caring for severely ill children at home pervades family life. Integrating the special care that the child requires with family life is often difficult. Of course, the experience varies with the child's condition, the family's circumstances, and the support available, but several themes are common. Some of the major effects on families of providing home care are shown in Table 2–1. We focus here on four main issues: the burden of daily care by families; social isolation

Table 2-1. Effects of Home Care on Families

Increased daily care responsibilities

Loss of control over daily life

Parents' isolation from extended family and friends

Disruption of sleep and social activities

Maternal depression

Interruption of patterns of usual child guidance

Child's social isolation

Parental neglect of ill child's sibling

Sibling's unresolved ambivalence toward ill child

Marital strain

Reorganization and renovation of living space

Lack of privacy

---

and the loss of control over daily life; the need for mutual support among families providing home care; and the stress on families.

The four issues affect families at different times and with different intensity. Families' adjustments seem to follow a variety of trajectories. For most, the first few months after the birth of a child with a significant and complex health problem, or after its diagnosis later in life, are an emotion-laden period (Burr, 1985). Many parents deny the severity of the problem or its extent at this time; others become angry with themselves, with the health care system, or with their child. The unpredictability of the child's course, seen in many situations, can add to family stress (Jessop & Stein, 1985). Parents' knowledge about their child's condition may be limited because information is lacking or poorly shared by professionals. Parents will often spend a great deal of time and effort tracking down information that will help them understand their child's condition and what they can do about it. Especially if they wish to bring their child home, they must develop caregiving skills and learn unfamiliar tasks. They must develop nursing skills, reorganize the home environment, adjust their social lives and employment, make arrangements with their other children, and seek support from extended families and friends. Many decisions must be made quickly at a time when the family is under great pressure.

Transitions are very important for children with severe illnesses and their families. Key transitions include the move from hospital or chronic-care facility to the community and home and the growth of children into adolescence and young adulthood. Transition from hospital to home can take place effectively but requires extensive planning and care and arrangements for follow-up of the discharge plan. Similarly, transition to young adulthood goes well for

most youngsters with severe illnesses. One father of a teenager with spina
bifida told us of the extra care required to determine which colleges that his son
was applying to were accessible to people in wheelchairs (Spina Bifida Association parent, personal communication, 1991). Teenagers face problems in
becoming independent from their families. As they reach young adulthood,
they often "age out" of important programs that provide support for children
with disabilities. The rules for eligibility for SSI benefits change during the
teenage years. Medicaid and Title V programs and state programs for specific
pediatric health conditions have upper age limits that suddenly curtail benefits
for these young people.

Feinberg (1985) delineates three stages in the adjustment of families to
home care: (1) the triumph of discharge; (2) six weeks to six months later,
when exhaustion and frustration with nurses and diminution of community
support set in; and (3) integration of the high-technology child into daily life
with the expectation of occasional problems with insurance companies, occasional incompetent nurses, medical crises, and rehospitalizations. Many families find that, after a year of intense struggle, they finally begin to understand
their limits and capabilities. They become knowledgeable about their child's
illness, often more so than most of the health professionals with whom they
interact (Anderson, 1985; Massie & Massie, 1976). They gain expertise in
managing the child's care and the panoply of providers. They learn to make
competent, skillful use of community resources.

Other families do less well in attaining an adequate level of self-care and
management capacity and need continuing support and guidance. A survey by
Quint and colleagues (1990) of 18 families providing home care to their
ventilator-dependent children found that the coping ability of primary caretakers, usually mothers, deteriorated as time passed. After two years, measures of family closeness and self-esteem from caring for their child had
diminished significantly. One can only speculate whether a more adequate
program of respite care, home nursing, and counseling would have prevented
these changes in families' ability to cope. For many families, home care goes
well except when there are significant transitions, such as the death of a
parent, the child's entry into school, or an exacerbation of the child's underlying health problem.

The Burden of Daily Care by Families

Families face relentless and consuming responsibilities of home care, constant
vigilance, restricted social life, and lack of time to meet personal and family
needs. The mother of Jennifer Marcos, a 9-year-old with severe asthma, said,
"You're not just a mother, but a nurse and doctor to this child 24 hours a

day.'' Mrs. Marcos has been unable to find a sitter willing to take on the responsibility of staying with Jennifer, and she wishes there were a baby-sitting cooperative for children with asthma (COPE). Similarly, VNS staff described the extraordinarily time-consuming care required by a 10-week-old infant severely ill with Pierre Robin syndrome. Each feeding alone takes two hours because of the baby's malformed jaw, tongue, and palate. The mother takes care of both the infant and her 18-month-old son while her husband works full-time. Until a respite-care nurse came to the home to administer the feedings, VNS had not appreciated the mother's exhaustion, anxiety, frustration, and need for relief (VNS). In another family, the complex feeding and medication regimens required by an infant with end-stage renal disease immobilized her 22-year-old single mother, and the child was hospitalized again until respite care could be provided (VNS).

Families caring for a severely ill child at home face a wide and often burdensome series of tasks significantly different from those faced by parents of apparently healthy children. The child may require special foods or unusual diets, equipment to aid breathing or feeding, and special vehicles to transport the child and the related equipment outside the home. At times, the home itself must undergo structural changes to improve physical access, bring in adequate electrical power, or provide space for home-care personnel. Parents must learn such new procedures as special feeding techniques and the care and cleaning of tubes in the child's stomach, intestine, urinary tract, veins, or breathing tract. Sophisticated devices that may be needed to monitor breathing, heart rate, or the concentration of chemicals in the blood require learning, attention, and time by parents.

Unquestionably, many parents experience emotional growth and enhanced self-esteem as they develop strength and competence in meeting the demands of home care. Marianna, a young single mother in the Einstein Pediatric Home Care program, spoke movingly of the confidence she has developed in learning to care for Luis, her severely disabled child. Holding out her hands, she said quietly, ''I can care for Luis myself—*with these hands.*''

SOCIAL ISOLATION AND LOSS OF CONTROL OVER DAILY LIFE

Families may require the emotional and physical support of extended family and friends. They need routine respite opportunities to maintain their equilibrium (Aday et al., 1988, p. 328; Feinberg, 1985; Prentice, 1986, p. 291; Ruben, 1982). Describing how it feels to cope alone with two daughters with von Willebrand's disease, Mrs. Abeson said eloquently and sadly, ''I feel like I am in prison'' (Hemophilia Center).

Some families rely on relatives, neighbors, and friends for help, but many others go it alone. Seven parents interviewed on one site visit are the primary caretakers of their chronically ill children and receive virtually no substantial help from family members or friends (Einstein). Only one mother had been able to teach a friend how to care for her child's tracheostomy. The extended family of another child refused to help care for the child because they are nervous and afraid. Most parents, especially those with the most severely ill children, have regrets but seem resigned to the reality of their sole respon- sibility for their child's care.

Family life and morale are thrown into imbalance by the unpredictability of the ill children's conditions (Jessop & Stein, 1985). Families may feel they have lost control over their daily lives. The likelihood of recurrent infections and repeat hospitalizations for children with many complex conditions— bronchopulmonary dysplasia, diabetes, cystic fibrosis, asthma, muscular dys- trophy, to name just a few—prevent families from planning ahead. Families providing home care rarely plan for trips and vacations (Thorp, 1987, pp. 74, 128), never knowing when an acute episode of illness will occur. "Planning events beyond those of today or tomorrow can seem pointless since the proba- bility of some unexpected crisis is always looming" (Feinberg, 1985, p. 38). Dependency on home-care personnel contributes to the feeling of loss of control. Thorp (1987) quotes the mother of a ventilator-dependent child whose experience typifies the frustration of needing many other people to provide care: "You have to sit and make phone calls all day, and then you sit by the phone and wait for people to call you back" (p. 126). Mothers report the confinement of having to plan errands around nurses' schedules (Thorp, 1987, p. 126).

Typically, sleeping schedules are disrupted (Burr et al., 1983). "One mother reported staying up three to four nights in a row because she had no night nursing coverage, and as a consequence she was too exhausted to carry on any routine daytime activity"; another said simply, "You never do sleep well" (Thorp, 1987, p. 125). Parents of children with tracheostomies find the fear of the child's inability to communicate especially disruptive; they "antici- pate their child having respiratory distress at night and being unable to call for help, and will therefore sleep in shifts or not at all" (Ruben et al., 1982, p. 638). Weary mothers of children with medically complex conditions often use the hours of daytime nursing coverage to sleep (VNS).

Many families experience isolation from friends, family, and community. Detailed descriptions of the daily schedules of mothers we interviewed at the Einstein Pediatric Home Care program were striking for one omission: No parent included personal time—to see friends, talk with a spouse, go to a movie, read a book. At the Regional Hemophilia Center the mother of two children with von Willebrand's disease talked about the social isolation created by the heavy demands of caring for her daughters. During the years when the girls had frequent episodes of bleeding, the mother could not leave them alone and had no friend, sitter, or family member who felt able to take responsibility for them for even a brief time. Now that the daughters receive home-administered care and are enrolled in school, the mother still leaves the house only rarely for brief errands because school staff fear that they cannot handle bleedings that might occur. Home-care responsibilities have greatly curtailed opportunities for daily contacts with friends and neighbors; consequently, the mother is thinking of buying a beeper so that she can be free from bondage to the telephone.

The majority of mothers of ventilator-dependent children in Thorp's study (1987) told her simply: "We don't go out." A single mother said of her social life: "No guy would go out with me." Fear of exposing their medically fragile children to contagious illnesses prevents many families from inviting friends to their homes or making visits. Ann Oster summarized the experience of caring for her son with chronic lung disease (1985): "The cornerstone of this experience is loneliness. Our family was isolated by the physical realities of hospitalization and therapy sessions, isolated socially by an experience that few other families share, isolated from each other by the crisis itself, with each family member needing to curl up somewhere for comforting" (p. 7).

Need for Mutual Support Among Families

Parent support groups appear to help with the isolation of caring for a chronically ill child. Mrs. Harnett, whose child with hemophilia is now a teen, feels that she received insufficient guidance in the early days. "Now I'm getting help, but I needed it earlier, to anticipate this teenage thing I've just been through. The opportunity to sit down with other parents wasn't available to me when Miles was small, or if it was, I didn't know it. Someone should have made more of an effort to get me involved. It would have been a great help if I could have picked up the telephone and talked to someone in the early years" (Hemophilia Center). Two Iowa mothers whose children have Goldenhar's syndrome and a severe, complex seizure disorder strongly expressed the need for support from other families with unusual conditions similar to those of their own children.

But professionals report that their efforts to establish support groups for parents or children meet with only minimal success. Obstacles have included problems of transportation, difficulties in getting babysitters, the low priority many parents place on verbal communication, and the perceived stigma of group membership. Families providing extensive home care may be unable to arrange for time away from their child. Family-initiated groups have had greater success, as evidenced by a group of mothers of children on renal dialysis who worked with the dialysis staff at one site to resolve a specific problem (Einstein).

A number of programs have experimented with different forms of parent-to-parent support. The Einstein Pediatric Home Care staff, recognizing the difficulties of maintaining ongoing group meetings of parents, is studying ways that staff can effectively relay information and ideas from one parent to another. The Family Friends program of the National Council on the Aging pairs older volunteers with families whose children have severe health impairments. Volunteers share with each other the successful actions of the families with whom they work, thereby transferring one family's experience to many others through their networks.

Stress on Families

The stress of living with a child's severe chronic illness takes many forms. According to Hobbs and colleagues (1985), serious long-term health impairment causes "what would be formally termed adjustment problems" in the ill children, their parents, and their siblings (p. 68). Caring for chronically ill children at home affects the adjustment of family members, marital relationships, and living arrangements.

Mothers' Adjustment

Parenting creates demands for all families, and depression is a frequent concomitant of raising children (McLanahan & Adams, 1987). But for parents of chronically ill children, the emotional lows may be greater than the usual uncertainty about a child's future. Anderson and Elfert (1989) found that the burden of care falls disproportionately on mothers of chronically ill children and that their needs as women become overshadowed by their children's needs. Depression is especially common among mothers of children with health impairments. Breslau and Davis (1986) found that mothers of chronically ill and handicapped children had significantly more depressive symptoms and onset at an earlier age than other mothers, although their depressive symptoms were no more profound than those of mothers of healthy youngsters. Similarly, Thorp (1987) found that depression commonly affects mothers of ventilator-dependent children.

Many mothers and professionals we interviewed confirmed the frequency of depression in caregivers, especially mothers, of children in home care. Symptoms were evident in caregivers as diverse as the Guyanan mother of a 15-month-old child with spina bifida in Queens, New York; the mother of a 16-

year-old with Werdnig-Hoffmann disease in the Bronx; the mother of a 6-year-old daughter with epidermolysis bullosa (a severe blistering skin disease) in rural Florida; the mother of two young daughters with von Willebrand's disease in Manhattan; and the Maryland mother of a 5-year-old daughter with a tracheostomy.

Supportive programs may, however, counter the prevalence of depression among caregivers. A study of excellent programs for children with developmental delay found that mothers of children enrolled in the programs had no higher incidence of depression than did other mothers. The mothers' feelings of well-being may be the result of participation in the programs (Dr. Jack Shonkoff, personal communication, 1990).

Children's Adjustment

Parents who care for severely ill youngsters at home face difficult challenges as they attempt ''to foster and facilitate growth and independence, necessary ingredients for healthy emotional development'' (Stein, 1987, pp. 27, 28). Chronic illness complicates these tasks of parenting, and children's psychological adjustment may suffer. Parenting is made more difficult by different patterns of growth and development, by concerns over proper discipline, and by different expectations parents may have for their child with a health impairment; yet services directed mainly toward the medical and surgical needs of the child may neglect parents' real needs for guidance in how to foster the child's development and psychological health. Mothers observe that the greatest deficiency in the services they receive is the lack of guidance concerning their children's growth and development (Burr et al., 1983; Pless & Pinkerton, 1975).

Although most children with severe illnesses develop and adjust well, others face serious problems. Studies in England, the United States, and Canada all indicate that a child with a chronic illness has about twice the likelihood of having a psychological or behavioral problem in comparison with a child without apparent illness (Cadman, Boyle, Szatmari, & Offord, 1987; Pless & Roghmann, 1971). Although in general most health conditions appear to create the same level of risk, children with conditions that affect the functioning of the central nervous system appear to face especially high risk (Breslau, 1985). As the youngsters get older, the symptoms persist, with great consequences for the children's life chances (Breslau & Marshall, 1985).

Several children whom we interviewed demonstrated severe emotional distress. A 16-year-old boy with hemophilia said, ''My mother has been a nervous wreck all my life.'' Like many other children with severe chronic illnesses, he feels smothered and overprotected. Despite being a good student, he was a truant for nearly a full school year and stayed with friends without informing his parents of his whereabouts, behavior at least in part a reaction to maternal overprotection (Hemophilia Center). A 14-year-old, 3-foot-tall boy with hypoplastic kidney disease since birth has had suicidal thoughts ever since he began dialysis several months earlier (Einstein). A 16-year-old boy in the Einstein Pediatric Home Care program whose body is severely twisted and shrunken by the ravages of Werdnig-Hoffmann disease and who was recently confined to bed and is respirator-dependent struggles with adolescent sexual feelings and fantasies with no physical relationship in which to express them.

Suicidal thoughts, feelings of social isolation, and being different from one's peers characterize many children with severe health impairments. Lack of friends and discrimination by peers are common experiences of these youngsters (Turner-Henson, Swan, & Holaday, 1991). A social worker-researcher in Chicago told us that every child she interviewed in a study of ventilator-dependent children reported suicidal thoughts (Illinois). She suspects that the death of at least one child in the study that was attributed to ventilator failure was, in fact, a suicide. Frates and colleagues (1985, p. 854) report that 17 of 54 ventilator-dependent children who were cared for at home over a 20-year period died, three from ventilator disconnection, but the researchers do not consider the possibility of purposeful self-destructive acts by any of the children. No home-care staff raised the issue of homicide in interviews with us. However, they readily acknowledge that child abuse and neglect and referrals of families to child protective agencies occur with some frequency among families with severely ill children at home (REACH, Einstein, VNS, and other sites).

Siblings

Home care affects not only parents and the ill child but also sisters and brothers. Many siblings benefit from having a health-impaired child at home. Families can be brought closer together (Burr et al., 1983, p. 1321), and older siblings can gain strength and competence from helping to provide care (Feinberg, 1985, p. 40). Siblings of children who are terminally ill with cancer and who die at home adapt better than do siblings of children who die in the hospital (Lauer et al., 1985). On the other hand, "Family life disruption is often felt most keenly by siblings" (Feinberg, 1985, p. 40). The tremendous demands placed on the time and energy of parents in caring for the ill child may leave little parental attention for the other children (Illinois; Ruben et al., 1982; Thorp, 1987).

The mother of Serena, a 9-year-old with severe cystic fibrosis, said that her greatest need is to be able to pay more attention to her 13-year-old son, whom she has neglected in order to provide the extensive care Serena requires

(COPE). The mother of a boy with hemophilia, deeply involved in his care for 16 years, said she has scarcely paid attention to her older son and has never attended his ballgames and band concerts (Hemophilia Center). Similarly, the mother of three children, including Anna, a difficult-to-manage 6-year-old with a severe seizure disorder, mental retardation, and autism, told us that her absorption in Anna's care causes her deep concern about Anna's 5-year-old sister, who has had to grow up quickly and now feels neglected, especially since the arrival of a new baby brother (Iowa). Feinberg (1985) observes, "Parents may valiantly strive to continue to attend the ballet recitals or football games of their other children. But the demands of the ill child or their own exhaustion make the continuation of these normal activities extremely difficult" (p. 38).

Siblings may feel angry, jealous of the sick child, and guilty about their own good health. Unable to verbalize their feelings and fears and affected by their parents' anxiety, they may experience emotional and behavioral difficulties (Ruben et al., 1982; Feinberg, 1985). Our visits with the families of Lorna, Terry, and Mary Ann illustrate these issues. The younger brother of Lorna, a child with cerebral palsy who suffered perinatal hypoxia and meconium aspiration and who died the week prior to our home visit, had been extremely attached to his sister. Ever since her death he has exhibited serious behavior problems in his Head Start class (REACH). The 8-year-old brother of Terry, a ventilator-dependent child cared for at home by his anxious parents, is prone to physical illness and is depressed and neglected. His mother is pregnant and the home-care staff are very concerned about the siblings' well-being (Maryland). Bobby, a 3-year-old whose 4-month-old sister, Mary Ann, has Down syndrome, has been difficult for the mother to manage ever since Mary Ann came home from the hospital. He has bitten Mary Ann, he yells a lot, and his mother is distraught because her previously well-behaved son disturbs his father, who is employed at night and must sleep during the day in their small, second-floor apartment. Bobby's mother is distressed that she cannot spend much time with Mary Ann on the exercises the physical therapist has prescribed. She has been unable to find a preschool program for Bobby, and the only break in his routine is occasional visits to an elderly neighbor (VNS).

Adolescents often deny problems in having ill siblings at home, but their experiences belie their denials. The healthy teenage sister of a ventilator-dependent child recounted her fears when, hospitalized for a lung abscess, she overheard the doctors say she might need a tracheostomy. She was terrified that she would end up on a ventilator like her sibling. For many adolescents, denial takes the form of unrealistic assessment of their responsibility for the ill child's care. One teenage brother of a respirator-dependent child responded to his parents' anxiety about ensuring care if they were no longer able to provide it by determining that he would leave junior high school, work, and care for his sibling (Illinois).

Marital Relationships

Marital relationships are strained for many families. Parents have little time to cultivate their own relationship. A study of parents providing home care of children with tracheostomies reports "a relatively high incidence of fathers leaving home at least temporarily after the child with the tracheotomy returned home from the hospital" (Ruben et al., 1982, p. 638). Many families we interviewed had experienced serious marital problems that they attributed in part to the demands of the child's illness. The mother of a teenager with hemophilia told of her absorption in caring for him since his hemophilia was diagnosed when he was 2 years old. The intensity of her involvement with her son virtually isolated her from her husband and the child's older brother; only now, when her child with hemophilia is ready to graduate from high school and live independently, is she facing the marital disruption that has been lying dormant for 14 years (Hemophilia Center).

Social workers attribute the disruption of marriages of parents with technology-dependent children to a constant stream of health workers in the home and a lack of privacy. Parents feel constrained from arguing or maintaining their sexual relationship (Illinois). The initial elation parents feel when they bring their ventilator-dependent children home from the hospital may be undermined by the toll that care assesses on their marriage (Aday et al., 1988, p. 327). When children with tracheostomies come home from the hospital, "Many times the child who was previously sleeping in his or her own crib or bed in another room is moved into the parents' room. Commonly, the father is displaced from the bed, or the room, or the child may begin sleeping with the mother. As one might well imagine, this is very disruptive to the parents' sexual relationship" (Ruben et al., 1982, p. 638).

The realignment of marital relationships brought on by caring for a medically complex child at home may be strengthening in some respects and disruptive in others. Feinberg (1985, p. 40) observes that "subtle marital discord" may occur in families of technology-dependent children. The mother as primary caregiver is often trapped in the impossible role of "superwoman," carrying out the jobs of mother, general manager, financial analyst, and personnel manager, while feeling unprepared for the responsibility; marital disruption is often a consequence (Illinois). Some mothers achieve competence and success in dealing with professionals, but their new-found strength may pose a threat to fathers who have previously been in control. Fathers often feel excluded from the child's care and resent the disequilibrium associated with the child's condition. A family therapist at the Ackerman Institute for Family Therapy, which provides counseling to families referred by the Regional Hemophilia Center at New York Hospital, described the mothers of children with hemophilia as "married to the medical care system"; these marriages to the system frequently supplant the parents' marriages to each other (Hemophilia Center).

Although parents express gratitude for the help that shift nurses provide, there are often unpleasant intrusions in marriage and family life. Over two-thirds of the families of ventilator-dependent children surveyed by Quint and colleagues (1990) felt that shift nurses invaded family privacy. Some nurses become over-involved with the family, discipline siblings and the ill child, disagree with the family about technical aspects of care, or disapprove of the family's life style (Illinois). Parents told one researcher, "We have people in and out all the time. You have to adjust to someone else's personality. . . . The hardest part is getting used to having all the people coming in. . . . You'd like to be able to walk nude to the shower or to have a fight with your husband" (Thorp, 1987, p. 137).

Family Living Space

Dependence on equipment and on the shift nursing necessary for the care of many children with complex medical conditions has dramatic effects on the physical setup within the home and on families' interactions. Feinberg (1985) describes the scene: "Nurses, other health care personnel, medical equipment, and suppliers can transform a home to that of a mini-intensive-care unit. Family members may feel as if they live in a medical fishbowl with the changing shifts, the routine resuscitations, the ringing of machine warning bells, and the frequent doctor appointments" (p. 38). Equipment breakdowns are inevitable. Every family in one study of ventilator-dependent children in home care experienced problems with equipment and vendors during the year before they were interviewed, several as many as 20 times (Quint, 1990).

Adequate electricity, lighting, and heat, sufficient electrical outlets and power, storage space for supplies and backup equipment, and access for partially immobilized children frequently require home renovations. Backup plans for emergencies must be arranged with ambulance services, police, fire departments, and highway patrols (Maryland). Discharge planning for a Maryland child with bronchopulmonary dysplasia entailed extermination of the rats and building a ramp at the back door of the home (Maryland). Sometimes the changes in physical arrangements are simpler but still emotionally disruptive. Parents told us about having to give away beloved family pets, removing favorite dust-catching stuffed animals, and giving up smoking before their children could come home.

Many families simply cannot afford to make their homes safe and suitable. Sarah Brown, a 9-year-old with severe asthma, sleeps in a hot Manhattan apartment because her parents cannot afford to buy the air conditioner that she needs (COPE). Some homes we visited—trailers in rural north Florida, walk-ups in New York City—were cold and crowded and lacked telephones, emergency exits, and transportation, in spite of parents' efforts to provide adequate arrangements for the ill child and the rest of the family (REACH and VNS). Sometimes the child's idiosyncratic needs create perpetual disruption. On one home visit, the television in the family's small apartment was blaring unmercifully; the nurse explained that, without the television, the 2-year-old with severe cerebral palsy, developmental delay, and hydrocephalus emits a constant, high-pitched shriek (REACH).

FUTURES FOR FAMILIES

Caring for a severely ill child at home offers extensive challenges to family life. What is remarkable is the resilience of children and families. Despite the many threats to the stability of the family and to the psychological health of parents and children, most youngsters do remarkably well and can become effective young adults. Similarly, the stamina and commitment of families in the face of frequent adversity and daunting demands on their resources are remarkable. These families depend greatly on community resources and efforts and on programs both federal and local. How well these efforts work for families greatly affects their abilities to cope.

Most families want their severely ill children to live at home. The demands they face are far from routine and beyond the caretaking responsibilities assumed by most families. The capability of families to manage the care of health-impaired children at home is highly sensitive to the functioning of the health care and education systems, the quality of services, and the financial costs and payment for care. The next chapters examine these elements of the social fabric and their implications for the ability of families to care for their chronically ill children at home.

3

The System of
Services for Families

John Jamison, a teenager with muscular dystrophy, is confined to a wheelchair. John requires nighttime oxygen therapy because his respiratory muscles, weakened by the ravages of the disease, cannot provide adequate oxygenation to his tissues without help. His sedentary life-style requires a special diet to prevent obesity. Mr. and Mrs. Jamison and John's brothers and sisters lift him from bed to wheelchair to toilet to breakfast table and then to specialized school transportation. The Jamisons receive psychological help to cope with John's feelings of being different from his friends and with the knowledge that his disease is uniformly fatal, although he may survive into young adulthood before succumbing to progressive lung failure. Physical therapy diminishes the painful contractures or locking of John's joints, and occupational therapy helps to keep him functional despite progressive muscle wasting. Modifications within the home permit wheelchair accessibility.

Wei Cheng, who survived a spinal cord injury, is paralyzed from the neck down. The upper centers of his brain work well, locking an effective mind in a body whose arms and legs and other parts function little or not at all. Wei requires nearly permanent attachment to a respirator and nursing care for eating and toileting. Physical and occupational therapy help to preserve what limited muscular function remains. During the flu season, a serious respiratory infection led to hospitalization because of the fragile nature of Wei's lung reserve. Community and educational services help Wei pursue intellectual growth and development.

Phyllis Volpi has osteogenesis imperfecta, a rare disease that makes her bones brittle and grow poorly. She needs specialized equipment in her home to prevent simple injuries from breaking her bones. Treatment for common childhood illnesses and some care for her bone problem and its consequences are provided near her home. Other services require Phyllis to travel many miles to see a bone surgeon, an eye doctor for the ocular complications that accompany the disease, and a respiratory specialist because the poor growth of her rib cage and supporting structures in her neck compromises breathing. Because Phyllis misses a lot of school, she needs help from her teachers and classmates so that she can keep up with her schoolwork. Her Scout leader has learned about Phyllis's disease and helps her and the other scouts adjust to her limitations.

Jimmy Tremaine, a child with bronchopulmonary dysplasia, depends on a ventilator and a great deal of other equipment in his home. Mr. and Mrs. Tremaine provide extensive home services for their son and rely on full-time home-based nursing as well. Jimmy requires careful monitoring of his medications. This is done by checking blood levels and looking for side effects; medicines keep his airways clear, yet these medicines make Jimmy sick to his stomach if given in too high doses.

SERVICES NEEDED BY CHILDREN AND FAMILIES

Consideration of these families' needs makes clear that home care entails far more than providing medicines, nursing care to change bandages, and special equipment. These children and their families are distinguished in two ways from those with acute, serious, but temporary illness, from children with major developmental problems, from other children with chronic conditions, and from other well children. First, these youngsters continually rely on specialized medical, nursing, educational, and community services over their lifetimes. Second, they receive extensive home-based treatments and therapies provided by either professionals or their parents. Failures in the medical and health care system are especially significant for these families because of their long-term, intensive involvement with and reliance on that system.

Care of a child with a severe long-term illness at home presents complex tasks that families whose children have no illness rarely face. The multiple services that families often need interact in ways that require coordination, and the changing intensity of caretaking activities calls for a continuum of services from acute hospital care to home care and integration into school and community life. Families providing home care for their severely ill children receive most services that they need, although the barriers they face often require vigorous advocacy, and the frequent lack of service coordination leads to conflicting advice and treatments.

Beyond often complicated medical and surgical care, these families require customized programs incorporating multiple services that allow them to care for their children at home. A home-care program for a child may involve nursing, physical and occupational therapy, nutrition services, respiratory therapy, and home educational services, among several others. Some children require intensive home nursing care, for up to 20 hours per day, to manage feeding tubes, respiratory care, or care of skin and healing bones. Nurses also help families to provide home care by increasing their knowledge of the illness, its treatment, and means of obtaining services. Effective nursing care includes not only direct treatments and procedures but also education and family support. Other treatments, such as respiratory, occupational, or physical therapy delivered at home, in school, or in health centers, may also improve the function of the child.

Help comes from several agencies—medical, nursing, home care, equipment suppliers, financing programs, schools, day-care programs, and nutritional services. Social workers may facilitate access to these services. Coping with a chronic illness increases the risk of psychological problems for both children and parents. Preventive mental health services that reinforce effective coping strategies and skills and improve understanding of and adjustment to illness may prevent the onset of psychological disturbance.

Children with special health care needs depend on the educational system to prepare them to meet the social, intellectual, and economic expectations of the adult community. Now that the large majority of children with severe chronic illnesses survive at least to young adulthood, it makes sense to consider their educational goals as preparation for adulthood rather than for early death as in years past. Schools fill both educational and socialization needs and are the link to other community activities and to the integration of the youngsters into community life. A few children must be home for lengthy periods or throughout their illness and their lives and must rely on home instruction, but most can attend school with special help. The usual patterns of learning and socialization cannot occur if the child is excluded from school attendance. A mother of a teenager with cystic fibrosis in Texas noted: "These children are trying to be normal while fighting for the recognition that they are not normal. There is no reason for these minds to go to waste just because they don't fit in the normal school mold. Chronically ill children have the same needs as other children— socially, emotionally, and educationally. They do have greater physical needs, but this shouldn't disqualify them for the other three" (Walker, 1986, p. 13).

Severely ill children present challenges to the educational system. For some, mobility impairment necessitates special schedules, transportation, or class placement. Others require extensive in-home tutoring because they are unable to be in school for prolonged periods. Young children with sensory deficits or developmental disabilities require early intervention that provides home teaching and trains parents to stimulate their children's development at home. In other cases, the matter may be as simple as educating the school about the child's condition so that he or she may participate in school activities without undue restrictions.

What is clear from stories of families whose children have highly complex medical conditions is their need for support from a variety of community-based services. Home care in this context encompasses comprehensive services and the support necessary to strengthen families' caregiving capacities, to prevent or overcome disability, and to improve the long-term functioning of both child and family. Beyond a comprehensive array of services, key elements for families include coordination of services, continuity among the different settings in which the child receives care, and a central role for families as the locus of care moves from hospital to home.

CURRENT SYSTEMS AND PROVIDERS OF SERVICE

Home- and community-based services for chronically ill children and their families are organized and delivered within four main service clusters: community-based home care and nursing services; hospitals and medical care; schools; and other community services. These four systems are complemented by community physicians and nurses, health departments, and a wide variety of providers of specialized therapies and equipment. Both the structure and the organization of each cluster affect the types and quality of services that families receive. Although most service programs operate in a competent manner, certain barriers limit families' access to needed services. And how effectively these four clusters integrate determines whether services are comprehensive, coordinated, and continuous.

Family needs merit a comprehensive and holistic view, yet services are typically narrow and leave many needs unmet. Hospital-based discharge planning may be thorough in medical terms, but neglect psychosocial care or educational planning. Plans may lack coordination with community health providers and nursing agencies, and careful planning for transition from one level of care to another is often absent. Schools may be unable to dispense medications called for in the plan or to provide programs for children who have frequent absences.

Community-Based Home Care and Nursing Services

Beyond families themselves, the central group of home-care providers is community nursing or home-care agencies, both public and private. Public health departments often have community nursing or home health care units. Visiting Nurse Associations in many communities offer home-based services for children and adults. Agencies vary greatly in size. Some provide a wide range of therapies, such as respiratory care, occupational and physical therapy, nutritional services, and speech and language programs along with more specific nursing care; others provide only direct nursing services. Most community nursing and home health agencies provide the bulk of their care to homebound elderly rather than to children. A few large agencies, such as the Visiting Nurse Service of New York, have departments dedicated to the home care of children. Given the lesser demand and relatively limited funding for in-home care for children, most agencies have few staff dedicated to child health care in the home. State regulation and licensure of these agencies are also highly variable, with widely disparate standards for staffing, personnel credentials, and monitoring.

Some financial support for home care for children with chronic illnesses flows from the Medicaid and the Title V Maternal and Child Health programs. Medicaid support, as described in Chapter 6, comes mainly through the direct benefit package and through waivers for home- and community-based care. Although predominantly a financing program, Medicaid has had some impact on home-care services, mainly by increasing the supply of community-based home-care agencies that would otherwise have no source of income for home-care for children.

Some additional funding for home-care programs comes from the federal–state Title V programs of Maternal and Child Health (MCH) and programs for Children with Special Health Care Needs (CSHCN). States have great latitude in determining the use of these funds (Ireys, Hauck, & Perrin, 1985), and some states use resources to provide care coordination. Nevertheless, few state Title V programs regularly provide home-care services; rather, support for CSHCN home-care programs has come mainly from time-limited grants. Many of the programs visited in this study received this grant funding, which has supported the development of these innovative activities but cannot provide the ongoing financial base for services.

Most home-care programs are freestanding; that is, they are separate from the health centers that provide specialty medical and nursing care for these children. In recent years, many hospitals and other large health care organizations (such as health maintenance organizations) have organized their own home health agencies, providing a stronger link from hospital care to home-based services. These developments reflect both diversification of hospital corporations to increase revenues and a desire on the part of health care organizations to have more control of the continuum of health services from inpatient to community-based care.

The struggle for adequate compensation constrains the quality and extent of home nursing care. Home nursing services are frequently limited to carrying out nursing procedures, mainly because payment is unavailable for care coordination, advocacy, or parent training. Private and public reimbursement usually covers only specific treatment procedures in the home. Changing dressings, maintaining respiratory equipment, delivering IV medications, and monitoring a gastrostomy (stomach) tube are important procedures that nurses carry out in homes and for which they receive payment from insurers. But teaching families what to expect about their child's illness and how best to monitor changes, helping families find other needed services, and interacting with teachers to integrate a child with special equipment or needing special procedures into school are equally important efforts that lack reimbursement.

Nurses with whom we met and their agency supervisors spoke frequently of their desire to teach families more about their children's care, but the mandate from those paying the bills was to do procedures rather than to teach. Where a family needed counseling in a crisis, help with referral to another agency, or education about the child's illness and its treatment, all tasks that many nurses do well, public and private insurers would not support these activities. And for some families, needed in-home services may have little to do with direct health care procedures. Some families need less intensive (and less costly) homemaker services, but their insurance policies cover only skilled nursing care. Their dilemma then is to do without essential services or to use skilled nurses to provide homemaking services under the guise of nursing procedures.

Hospitals and Medical Care

Many families begin their experience with the child's severe long-term illness through a hospital stay when their youngster's health condition is diagnosed and treatment is begun. These hospitalizations are often prolonged and cause various degrees of separation between child and family. Many children, as their condition grows more acute, experience frequent, additional stays in a hospital. Hospitals for these children and their families have a central place in their lives and in influencing the cost of their care.

Most specialized health services are provided through tertiary-care hospitals with comprehensive pediatric departments. The staffs include specialists in pediatric medicine and surgery. Most such centers are equipped with up-to-date technologies and provide an extensive array of diagnostic, treatment, and laboratory services, often in association with research on specific childhood health conditions. Many programs are in general hospitals or children's hospitals affiliated with nursing and medical schools.

Many specialty hospitals have regional centers for children with specific diseases such as hemophilia, arthritis, and cystic fibrosis that provide a range of high-quality medical and surgical care, although other support services may be absent. The child with hemophilia may see a multitude of health providers (pediatricians, hematologists, orthopedists, and blood bank specialists) but is less likely to have help with psychosocial needs relating to hemophilia and its complications and with educational planning related to frequent brief absences from school.

Most hospitals organize children's health services around specialty programs that treat organ systems, such as children's kidney or heart programs. The programs provide sophisticated, intensive care for a discrete set of illnesses and emphasize specialized medical and nursing services. Programs may coordinate care for health conditions that require attention from several health-related disciplines, so that a child with spina bifida, for example, may receive services from a neurologist, neurosurgeon, urologist, specialized nurse, and physical and occupational therapists, among others. Some programs, especially those that receive support from disease-specific voluntary associations (for example, the Muscular Dystrophy Association, the Juvenile Diabetes Foundation, and the Cystic Fibrosis Foundation) or from the federal Bureau of Maternal and Child Health for specialty programs (for example, Pediatric Pulmonary, Hemophilia, and Juvenile Arthritis Centers), provide extensive multidisciplinary care, including social services, educational specialists, and psychological services. This breadth of multidisciplinary services depends almost entirely on these federal or voluntary association sources of funding. As described in Chapter 6, health insurance reimburses poorly for the broader array of services.

Because of the complex nature of many of the health conditions that require home-care services, few of the specialized health services that these children require are provided outside of comprehensive medical centers. Most children have a community-based health provider, either a physician or a nurse, although the roles of community professionals in caring for these children are often ill-defined (Kanthor et al., 1974; Okamoto & Shurtleff, 1981; Iowa). Parents can be confused about whom to call for advice about a fever or a change in the child's eating habits. And the emphasis on specialized medical services may leave many severely ill youngsters underimmunized or lacking screening for more common conditions that are part of the general health care provided to most other children. Linking hospital services to these community-based services represents an important task in the management of these children with severe illnesses.

Lack of a community treatment base requires families to travel to a central unit for many services. The child who needs occupational or physical therapy may be expected to return to the centralized center, often at great inconvenience to the family. Yet many therapies can be provided closer to home by training less specialized therapists to meet the needs of that child.

Specialty health centers face disincentives to decentralizing their programs and offering services at the community level where most children live and receive home care. Hospital-based centers that treat children from a wide geographic area are poorly informed about services in the many communities that refer children to them. Centralized health centers have difficulty maintaining the linkages with home- and community-based services that are essential to families. Transitional hospital programs exist in a few communities, providing key links between specialty centers and community-based services (Merkens, 1991).

Centralized care centers, nevertheless, provide important benefits. They allow the development of expertise in the variety of complications, treatments, and outcomes for the individually rare conditions that children have. Development of such knowledge and skills requires the centralization of highly specialized services and investigations. The tasks facing centralized health centers are to coordinate effectively with community-based services and to collaborate as part of a broader system of care for children who live in communities. Such a collaborative system allows greater flexibility with the changing nature and intensity of the child's illness at different points in his or her life and improves the integration of the child and family into the community.

That medical specialization, while improving technical aspects of care, has increased the fragmentation of services is well recognized (Lewis & Sheps, 1983). Over ten years ago, Pless, Satterwhite, and Van Vechten (1978) reported that medical care of children with complex medical conditions such as juvenile rheumatoid arthritis and spina bifida exhibits "a pattern whereby basic care is either divided or duplicated, but with many of the supportive aspects of care neglected in a high proportion of families . . . such patterns are typical of most children with chronic disorders" (p. 9). Continuity of care for such children is the main determinant of families' satisfaction with specialty care (Breslau & Mortimer, 1981) but is lacking for many of them.

Emphasis on specialization allows families access to up-to-date technologies and information about common and uncommon complications of their child's condition. But specialization means that less attention is given to issues that allow families to provide home care: direct family support services, modifications of the home environment to improve home care, education about the illness and elements of self-care, and psychological help to improve coping skills. The comprehensive task of caring at home for a child with complex health needs requires a comprehensive response (American Academy of Pediatrics, 1986).

Discharge planning is one of the services that comes to the forefront for children who need complex care at home. Families and professionals told us frequently that, when children with complex illnesses are discharged from the hospital, parents often feel that no one is following up. They feel alone in the trenches. A Children's Home Health Network survey of over 100 doctors who work with ventilator-dependent children found that neither physicians in the discharging hospitals nor those in the community were clear about who was in charge (Illinois).

Health care is also provided in a variety of community settings, including public health departments, private pediatric and family practices, and agencies offering specialized therapies, such as speech and hearing services. Health-impaired youngsters and their families utilize these community-based health and medical services, sometimes in conjunction with the specialized care they receive from specialty medical centers and home health agencies. For many families with severely ill children, information on these services can be hard to find.

In some communities, primary-care pediatricians are unwilling to care for complex, chronically ill children, referring them instead to specialty health services out of the community. In other communities it has been difficult to enroll pediatricians in programs that attempt to decentralize the care of children to the community level, especially if the children are covered by Medicaid. Community-based physicians who feel unqualified to manage the care of chronically ill children receive little training and support from the specialty centers.

From the viewpoint of the community physician, lack of help in providing services to children with unusual diseases, lack of support from the specialty center, and lack of education and resources make the task more difficult. Further, inadequate compensation for cognitive services, care coordination, and education of parents is a disincentive for community providers to become involved in a serious and satisfactory way with these children and their families.

Schools: Public Education in the Least Restrictive Environment

Important federal legislation assures access to education for children with handicapping conditions. Public Law 94–142, the Education of the Handicapped Act of 1975 (EHA), assures a free and appropriate public education in the least restrictive environment to children with handicaps. This act, renewed and expanded by Public Law 99–457 and renamed as the Individuals with Disabilities Education Act (IDEA) in 1991, mandates special education services throughout the United States and encourages a multidisciplinary approach to problems that interfere with a child's educational progress. The expansions of the act also provided incentives to identify children with disabilities in the first three years of life.

Most children who receive services through IDEA have problems in how they learn: Youngsters with speech impairments, learning disorders, and mental retardation account for 3.5 million (about 85 percent) of the total number of children served under this act (U.S. Department of Education, 1987). IDEA has a category of other-health-impaired that includes children with long-term health problems. The original regulations defining children's eligibility for services listed specific examples of health conditions that could interfere with the child's educational progress under the other-health-impaired category. These examples included tuberculosis, asthma, sickle cell anemia, hemophilia, and leukemia. Between 1985 and 1986, some 50,000 children in this category received services. As IDEA has been implemented, this small category, unlike the larger groups of children with learning impairments, generally includes youngsters who have impairments of mobility or other medical problems but who have normal cognitive abilities and no special problems in their ability to learn.

The special services that are available under IDEA are of major importance to young people who have severe health impairments and can make it possible for children to stay on track in school. Special transportation, physical therapy, medication administration during the school day, home or hospital instruction during an illness that prevents regular school attendance, psychological services, and modified physical education are just some of the services to which eligible youngsters may be entitled. The additional demands on school districts vary widely. Especially for small or significantly underfunded districts, financial demands can be severe and create difficult choices among competing priorities—extensive services for relatively few children or basic services for all children.

Section 504 of the Rehabilitation Act, another piece of civil rights legislation, prohibits discrimination in public facilities against people with disabilities. This legislation has been the basis for legal action to improve access to public school settings of children with chronic illnesses. Unlike Public Laws 94–142 and 99–457, however, Section 504 provides no direct funding to state or local education authorities to meet the statutory obligations. Therefore, it has been less effective in stimulating development of programs to assure access than have been the special education laws.

Children gain access to special services at school through the development of an Individual Educational Plan (IEP), a formal document that sets forth the particular services that the school will provide to the child. In developing the plan, the school staff evaluates the student's special needs. Once drawn up, the plan must be approved by the child's parent or guardian. The provision in the regulations related to parental approval of the IEP is a key element in supporting the rights of families. Parents who disagree with the IEP's provisions have specific rights and protection through grievance procedures that are rarely available in other agencies.

Severe illness affects children's learning in several ways (Table 3–1). It may directly impact cognitive functioning and change the child's capacity to learn. Some conditions are associated with delays in development, although most have no apparent direct effect on cognitive abilities. Medications, such as those for asthma or seizures, may affect a child's learning abilities or diminish the child's alertness. Illness may increase fatigue and make the child unable to work as consistently as his or her classmates. Frequent medical care visits and occasional hospitalizations increase school absence, as do the times when the child is bedridden at home.

IDEA appropriately focuses on special education and the needs of the large number of children with impairments in their ability to learn. Special education programs have focused on meeting the learning needs of these students. In contrast, children with complex medical conditions in the "other health impaired" category fit less well into special education. These children, often with normal cognitive abilities, rarely require special education classroom settings and are best served in regular education classes (Mearig, 1985).

School systems struggle to provide services to children with severe illnesses. Their needs for such specialized health services as the management of devices in schools (for example, respirators, feeding tubes, tracheostomies, or urinary catheters), dispensing medications, special emergency policies, or special diets create complicated tasks for schools facing difficult choices with limited resources.

Table 3-1. Classification of Childhood Long-term Health Conditions and Effects in Learning

Effects	Conditions
Conditions that *may* affect cognition directly:	Complex craniofacial anormalies (e.g., Pierre Robin syndrone) Spina bifida Major seizure disorders
Conditions that *may* affect cognition through side effects of treatment:	Leukemia Bronchopulmonary dysplasia
Conditions with little or no cognitive impact:	Arthritis Cystic fibrosis Hemophilia Tracheostomy or ventilator use

Children receiving home-care services may have inadequate assessment of their developmental and educational needs. In the context of planning for nursing services, specialized therapists, diets, and equipment, careful assessment of the impact and implications of the child's health condition on schooling may be forgotten. "Not all [families] felt as secure in the knowledge of the developmental and educational needs of their children. Presumably, the complexity of medical management meant that less attention was focused on developmental issues. Consequently, few parents brought their children home with an educational plan, and most of the children had not received developmental assessments to clarify their educational and social needs" (Burr et al., 1983, p.1322). Similar findings come from the community studies of Pless, Satterwhite, and Van Vechten (1978).

Chronic illness affects a child differently at each stage of development. A child born with a severe health problem and a teenager who develops a major physical disability at age 15 face different tasks of adjustment. Understanding the developmental impact at each age and especially how the health condition may impede education and development is essential to planning for these children and their families. Especially for very young children, assessment of developmental impact and involvement with early intervention programs can improve the child's long-term outcome and strengthen the ability of family members to learn ways of improving their child's development at home as well (Magrab, 1985; Meisels & Shonkoff, 1990).

Three aspects of school programs remain particularly problematic for children receiving extensive home-care services: access to health services in school, educational services at home, and vocational planning (Hobbs, Perrin, & Ireys, 1985; Shayne, Walker, Perrin, & Moynihan, 1987). These are discussed below.

Access to Health Services in School
Some children with severe chronic illnesses require specialized equipment during the school day and special transportation to and from school, while others without need of special equipment require medication during the school day. Children who depend on respirators or other equipment in school may require nurses or other attendants to assist with the equipment. Schools are at times reluctant to enroll these children. As some researchers observe:

Generally, schools will not permit a child with a tracheostomy in the classroom unless there is a full-time registered nurse in attendance. This nursing situation exists in New York City only in programs for multiply handicapped children. For non-mentally handicapped school-age children, there are several other alternatives: (1) home tutoring, which is definitely inadequate for purposes of socialization and generally inadequate educationally because the time is so limited; (2) parent or guardian accompaniment in the classroom, which is not a feasible alternative for families with younger children and a questionable alternative from the perspective of socialization as well; or (3) special arrangements whereby the parent assumes responsibility for the tracheostomy by being "on call" to the school in case of an emergency. (Ruben et al., 1982, p. 639)

Schools may look askance at nurses accompanying children to school and riding the school bus, and the presence of the child's special equipment in the classroom and the need for special procedures in the case of a medical emergency. (Feinberg, 1985, p. 41)

The increasing number of children attending school who depend on technologies has led to development of guidelines for their management in educational settings. The most extensive guidelines are those prepared by Project School Care at the Boston Children's Hospital. They describe health procedures for schools (for example, tracheostomy care, management of feeding tubes, and urinary catheterization) and set forth recommendations for types and training of personnel to provide care in the schools.

Children with chronic illnesses need medication during the school day, yet many schools lack means of dispensing medications. We learned of a 6-year-old with severe asthma whose mother goes to school daily to give the child medication since there is no school nurse to dispense it, despite the fact that the teacher and principal are extremely understanding about the child's asthma (COPE). Most schools have limited school health services, especially on a full-time basis. Elementary schools, which are typically smaller than secondary schools, often lack regularly available school health personnel. The youngster who routinely needs medication must either be restricted to the small number of schools that have full-time health personnel or receive medication through another mechanism.

Requiring a student to be in a setting with full-time health personnel restricts that child's access to community-based education in the least restrictive environment. In general, children can be better served through implementation of medication policies that define the personnel in each school who can dispense medications and provide those individuals with training and supervision from health personnel elsewhere in the system. As children develop their own self-care skills, they should be able to take their own medications.

Educational Services at Home
Home instruction at best offers a pale substitute for schoolroom education and at worst is inaccessible to many severely ill children. Many school systems require two to four weeks of consecutive absence before providing home instruction, yet most chronically ill youngsters have frequent absences of

shorter duration. Even when available, home-based education is typically limited to a few hours each week, during which the youngster must receive instruction in all of his or her courses: science, math, language, social sciences, and English. Some school districts have registries of children with chronic illnesses. When the children are absent, they immediately become eligible for home instruction services. These programs aim to return youngsters to school as soon as possible, for both education and socialization. They encourage classmates to visit with the child at home when school absence becomes lengthy.

Vocational Planning

Finally, vocational counseling, a service needed by many children with severe long-term illnesses, is rarely available. The New York Hospital Regional Hemophilia Center is an exception, providing early counseling to elementary-school children and helping teenagers make career choices consistent with their health conditions. Many illnesses prevent achievement in certain vocations, but most children can in fact become productive adults. Vocational training is essential to their effective participation in adult society.

Other Community Services

The intensity of service needs for most children with severe illnesses changes over time. Crises require acute, high-technology, in-hospital services; at other times, home services are needed. Many services such as respite programs, rehabilitation programs, and specialized day care fall along the continuum. Respite and day-care services are desperately needed but typically unavailable. There are few pediatric skilled nursing facility beds or group homes for medically complex children. Even foster care placement is difficult.

The lack of a continuum of services between hospital and home means that many families have no viable alternatives to home care. As a program director said, "Parents are told 'Here's your option. It's home or home.'" (Maryland). From the view of adolescents, the alternatives to home care are few. An adolescent told us, "People could leave their homes if there was a place where they could live, like living with Mom, but not with Mom, where we could grow up and develop ourselves" (Hemophilia Center). Attention to these transitions, from hospital to home, from childhood to young adulthood, and from chronic-care facility, rehabilitation programs, and respite services to home are needed.

Most communities provide a cluster of social support services. Some services are geared to the needs of special populations, including children with chronic illnesses, while others serve the general population. Many services play important roles for children and families simply by enabling families to participate in normal, regular, community life. Children with chronic health conditions require not only specialized services; they also need ready access to services such as recreational programs, community center activities, and Girl Scouts and Boy Scouts in which all children participate. Some programs make provisions to ensure the inclusion of health-impaired children. For example, some Scout troops adapt their programs so that children with severe health limitations can join. However, in general, gaining access to community-based programs that serve the general population of youngsters is problematic for chronically ill children, and efforts are needed to ensure that these children and their families are served.

Day care, essential to many families' economic self-sufficiency, is a much-needed community service that families with health-impaired children report difficulty in obtaining. Although some programs accommodate children with complex medical conditions, most are unwilling or unable to assume responsibility for their care. Some exemplary programs have developed to meet the growing need for child care. Handicare, a day-care program in Iowa City, accepts 60 children with severe health conditions whose developmental level is up to first grade. It is remarkable for its special organization of "classes" for children. Youngsters are grouped for each activity by their specific developmental level in social, physical, and cognitive areas. For example, a child with spina bifida with normal intelligence plays with his or her age peers for learning and social activities but is grouped with younger children for outdoor play. This program, founded by a woman who saw an unmet need for children with severe illnesses, underscores what can be accomplished when people with determination act.

Prescribed Pediatric Extended Care centers (PPEC) are day health care programs whose services are prescribed by physicians and therefore qualify for insurance reimbursement. This program in Tampa, Florida, offers day medical care in a group setting instead of hospitalization or home care. For parents, PPEC provides day care, respite, and special training in the care of their children. For children, PPEC offers a group experience that removes them from the isolation of their homes and allows them to interact with peers (Pierce, Lester, & Fraze, 1991).

Most compellingly, families relate time and again the importance of respite care. Adequate respite care can decrease the long-term dependence on public institutions and thereby be a cost-effective investment (Brimblecombe, 1974). Respite care may be especially important in maintaining vulnerable home-care programs during family transitions or crises. Opportunities for relief from the constant demands of caring for severely ill children allow households to regroup and often renew resources. Respite care can take many forms, including day-care services, in-home services, or even overnight camps. Nevertheless, most communities lack opportunities that provide time off for families from the strenuous and continuing care of a severely ill child.

In larger metropolitan areas, chapters of disease-oriented voluntary associations may offer support groups for families whose children have a particular health condition such as cystic fibrosis, hemophilia, or diabetes. These associations may also provide financial assistance for such equipment as wheelchairs. However, many of these organizations emphasize research rather than support services, and availability of the programs varies greatly from community to community. In impoverished rural areas and inner cities, where basic social institutions have crumbled, the lack of access to services presents especially grave challenges.

Child welfare services, both public and private, provide child protective services, foster care, and specialized adoptions when families are unable to care for their own youngsters. Professionals in the programs visited perceive that children with severe health problems are at greater risk of child abuse and neglect than other children and that referrals to child welfare agencies are sometimes necessary. Family service agencies and community mental health centers also offer individual and group counseling for parents and children. These agencies can be especially helpful when counselors understand the particular issues raised by children's chronic illnesses.

CHANGING NEEDS: COORDINATION AND THE CONTINUUM OF CARE

Fragmentation of Care: Lack of Coordination

Children often receive piecemeal services. A child may get comprehensive in-home therapies but have inadequate resources to maintain educational progress. Needs may change over time, but the system of services may be inflexible and insensitive to changing needs. Efforts to coordinate appointments, providers, and conflicting treatment demands are frustrating for parents who often have little understanding of the maze of services. Coordination of care is essential for families whose children receive care from many providers.

Sometimes families are the scapegoats for problems that originate with poor coordination and communication. Andy Madison, a 10-year-old who had cardiac surgery shortly after birth, has had worsening problems for the past five years. Sharp pain, circulatory problems in his legs, one shortened leg, chronic fatigue, and a clotted vein in his abdomen sent him to numerous physicians, without change in his condition. Andy's parents have become extremely frustrated that no one seems able to help him; if a treatment plan exists, they do not understand it. Because the parents have become a squeaky wheel in the medical care system, they have the reputation of being hostile and demanding. Yet careful coordination with the parents could have prevented most of the problems (REACH).

Care coordination or case management integrates treatment and monitoring into a family-based plan. The plan provides for the long-term growth and development of the child and the support of family needs over time. The coordinator of care assures access to services needed by families, helps the family resolve conflicts among plan elements, encourages communication among providers and between providers and family, and assists to educate families about resources and about illness. Currently, many families coordinate their own care, yet for most families, especially in early phases of illness when they are relatively unsophisticated about the care system and the array of helping resources, coordinating care can be a difficult task. Needs go unaddressed even though good resources may be nearby. Parents may find one therapist suggesting one approach to a certain problem and another recommending an entirely different approach. A care coordinator can improve the knowledge base on which families make decisions and help them to understand the decisions better.

Parent advocates agree that a key goal is to enable families to develop their own skills and provide coordination of care for their own children and households. Nevertheless, often at the initiation of home-care services and for several months thereafter, at times of key transition within the household, or for households with great need or limited resources, care coordination by individuals outside the family may be essential.

Several models of care coordination by those outside the home currently exist. Most rely on nurses, but others have used lay community counselors, social workers, or physicians to provide these services. In an important demonstration, Pless and Satterwhite (1972) showed that lay counselors with minimal training can provide advocacy and coordination to families with children who have a wide variety of chronic illnesses. More recent demonstrations using nonprofessional individuals who live in the communities they serve suggest that this model may effectively provide care coordination without needing to rely upon less available and more costly professionals.

Lack of coordination affects many families. Although specialty health centers may provide high-quality, comprehensive, even multidisciplinary services, they often neglect coordination with families' primary care and community-based services. The specialty health center may, for example, choose to have mental health services provided on-site rather than in the parents' community, even though satisfactory services exist closer to the individual family's home. Lack of coordination with the primary care level means that a family either must travel great distances from its home to the specialty center or must utilize community health providers who know little about the child's condition, history, and basic health care plan. Even within medical centers, where multiple specialties are involved, lack of coordination frequently occurs. The family may see one specialist one day and another the next. Inadequacies of medical record systems mean that information gathered by one professional is shared only with difficulty with another. Incentives to develop effective teamwork are limited.

For children with complex, long-term health care needs, the sheer number of providers with whom the children and families interact can itself be a source of frustration and strain. Betsy Anderson (1985), the mother of a child with spina bifida, observed: "Families must learn to deal with very complex systems of health and social services. . . . There are many more providers of services on the scene. . . . [and] a lack of mandates or incentives for many services systems which impinge upon children and families to coordinate and collaborate their activities" (pp. 3–8). Thorp (1987) affirms, "Unless there is interdisciplinary collaboration in supporting home care for the technology assisted child, the family becomes the victim of the many professionals who should be helping. Burdens may be inadvertently increased" (p. 47).

Families experience many difficulties in dealing with the various providers their children need. For example, arranging visits to clinics that meet on different days of the week can require several trips to the hospital and cause repeated absences from school. A family in rural Florida expressed anger that their 10-year-old, whose severe heart disease requires care in several clinics at the tertiary care center in Gainesville, had missed untold school days over the years because providers were unable to consolidate clinic visits on a single day (REACH). Waiting in hospital emergency rooms with a seriously ill child can be frightening. The mother of a 13-year-old with severe asthma in Manhattan described the long, harrowing hours of waiting for care for her son's asthma attacks and her own difficult process of learning finally to speak up and get attention for him (COPE).

Parents report, too, that it is common to receive contradictory advice from different physicians or other providers who treat their children. One family feels caught between the physician's insistence that their 8-year-old son, who has a brain tumor and a tracheostomy, is too ill to attend school and the nurse-coordinator's and school's assessment that the child should attend (Maryland). Similarly, the depressed, mentally slow mother of a 16-month-old with developmental delay has made numerous trips to doctors' offices from her fifth-floor Queens walk-up to obtain a prescription for the orthopedic shoes that have been insistently recommended by the physical therapist; the pediatrician and orthopedist cannot agree on which physician should write the prescription

(VNS). Families' irritation with contradictory professional advice and byzantine clinic schedules, when it persists over months and years, can escalate and interfere with care.

An additional factor that complicates families' interactions with service providers is the fact that many services are accessed through an array of private and governmental organizations. Parents "must learn about resources in their community and deal with many bureaucracies with special rules relating to eligibility for health and social services" (Stein, 1987, p.27). In addition to hospitals and insurance companies, parents deal with state Medicaid agencies, Title V Services for Children with Special Health Care Needs programs, nursing agencies, equipment vendors, public assistance departments, social service organizations, and even fire, police, and emergency medical departments. Many parents are not prepared to deal with the bureaucratic maze. Thorp observes that taking on the role of managing the child's care, negotiating with providers, accessing nursing care, supplies, and equipment, and arranging for payment may be especially difficult for parents who have been in a relatively helpless role during their child's hospitalization, when a team of skilled professionals has carried out these tasks (Thorp, 1987, p. 36). Marianna, the young, single mother of both Luis, a 5-year-old with severe asthma, and 2-year-old Marco, described her social services "system." A resident of the South Bronx, this mother has a "general social worker" who is affiliated with the Human Resources Administration through which the family gets AFDC welfare benefits and a home attendant for Luis. A caseworker from the family agency helps her with access to the Kennedy Developmental Center program where she has another social worker for Luis and still another social worker for little Marco. Luis receives Supplemental Security Income (SSI); thus he has a social worker from the Social Security Administration. Luis attends TOTS, a preschool program, where he has still another social worker/counselor (Einstein).

Perhaps most neglected is coordination with agencies outside the medical arena. Social services, early intervention programs, schools, community recreation programs, and day-care services typically rely mainly on parents' information without direct communication with the specialty health providers for the child. Such coordination may appear trivial to some; however, this lack of coordination often means that youngsters are excluded from appropriate school opportunities despite their abilities to compete effectively in educational programs. Or day care may be denied because a provider is worried about the liability or health risks associated with including a child with severe long-term illness. Thus, coordination can be a stimulus for the effective integration of the child into his or her community.

Interest in the concept of care coordination is expanding swiftly. The notion of coordinating care for children with special health needs was a key concept in early work of the Children's Bureau when it was directed by Martha May Eliot. The concept remained in embryonic form until the past decade. Today there are numerous informational and planning conferences, and a variety of health, social, and community agencies have what are called "case managers" or "care coordinators." Ironically, some families face not only a wide variety of competing and at times conflicting community agencies, but even five to ten case managers, thus perpetuating the fragmentation of services. What is needed is one person to be the care coordinator for the family.

CENTRAL ROLES FOR PARENTS

Parent advocates believe that a fundamental flaw in the American health care system is the exclusion of parents. Betsy Anderson (1985) observes that parental input into health care lags behind that in other systems, especially education. "The traditional view of the patient, and family by extension, has been as a passive recipient of care. . . . That passive role, which may have a limited place in some acute care situations, is now recognized as inappropriate for those individuals with chronic disabilities whose involvement with the medical system will generally be lifelong" (pp. 4–8). Denial of opportunity for families and children to play major roles in managing their own care sends families these messages:

1. The value of the contributions families and individuals can make is negligible. 2. Professionals know best and can handle it all. In fact, if they are not doing it, then it must not be important. 3. People with disabilities and their families get in the way and slow down the process. They are part of the problem, not part of the solution. (Anderson, 1985, p. 15)

Clearly, parents look to health and medical professionals, especially physicians and nurses, not only for technical care but also for emotional support, training in care, and understanding of their children's conditions and needs. Many providers and parents establish satisfying relationships, with parents finding support and solace in the partnership with professionals. Thorp (1987) found that mothers reported that professionals had been helpful to them (p. 163), and nurses and physicians were the professionals who were mentioned most frequently as helpful. Yet the most pervasive and sensitive issues in the relationship between parents and professionals, from the families' perspective, are the participation of families in, and control of, care and emotional support. The mothers in Thorp's (1987) study, while reporting support from health care providers, also experienced significant problems. One-third of the mothers "reported feeling it was difficult for doctors to take their perspective. Said one, 'They have no idea how hard it is.' Said another, 'What needs to happen most? Educate the doctors. They need to be educated in family needs'" (p. 136).

Ann Oster, whose child was born prematurely and is ventilator-dependent, describes her family's experience during the first several years of her son's life: "Many of our contacts with professionals were destructive to our self-esteem" (Oster, 1985, p. 6). Oster's involvement with other families has led her to observe the frequency of such experiences among parents of children with conditions similar to those of her son Jimmy. Professionals are often insensitive to parents, failing to provide the information and emotional support that parents of newly diagnosed, seriously ill children crave (Oster, 1985, pp. 6–7). Poor and poorly educated parents often feel vulnerable to decisions made by physicians without their knowledge. One such mother, whose child with severe asthma had a playground accident that led to a colostomy, told us angrily about a psychiatrist appearing in her child's hospital room to interview him, without her prior knowledge and consent (COPE). In New York, the mother of a child with asthma succinctly summarized parents' complaints about health and medical providers: "Medical people sometimes do not deal well with families and children" (COPE).

We met many families in exemplary home-care programs who have learned to take charge of their children's care. When parent empowerment is the goal, the results can be impressive, even in the face of enormous obstacles. Marianna, the South Bronx single parent with two children and seven social workers, talked almost with disbelief about her newly acquired ability to manage not only her child's care but also her own life. "I feel so good about myself now," she said (Einstein). Mrs. Bates, whose child's asthmatic condition was complicated by the playground injury that led to a colostomy, spoke with delight of learning at last to manage the doctors instead of having them manage her (COPE). A pulmonary subspecialist said admiringly that parents who have learned through the home-care program to speak up to the medical providers are better advocates for their children, whose care improves as a result. Some physicians may dislike being challenged, he said, but ultimately, parents who are assertive and informed make the physician's job much easier (Einstein).

Most families can learn to become the coordinators of their own child's care. As Anderson (1985) points out, the long-term care of the child in the home is predominantly the family's responsibility and, although family members may have only limited decision making in initial phases of hospitalization, they ultimately take on responsibility for their child at home, just as other parents do. Like all other families, they may need help through transition and education and advice to hone their skills. But they mostly need information with which to make more informed decisions.

PROGRAMS THAT HELP

Programs across the country effectively provide important parts of the services that families with severely ill children need. In the Bronx, New York, nurse-practitioners, pediatricians, and families develop lasting bonds that diminish the psychological and social impact of long-term illness in children and provide services at every level from home to hospital. The Pediatric Home Care program at the Albert Einstein College of Medicine assures that children and their families facing a serious long-term childhood illness have the best possible outcomes. The program enrolls families whose children have a wide variety of chronic long-term illnesses, including spina bifida, sickle cell disease, and severe asthma. The program operates from an institution that has an ethos of supporting families. Pediatric Home Care enables families to take increasing responsibility for the care of their own child by maximizing integration of health, educational, and social services, especially at the home level (Stein, 1987).

Iowa's Mobile and Regionalized Child Health Specialty Clinics for children with special health needs offer comprehensive services to youngsters with varied and complex health conditions. Nurses collaborate with educators who have special education backgrounds, coordinate services with families, and find resources at the community level. These regional systems enable Iowa's rural population to obtain the majority of services close to home rather than traveling great distances to major health centers hundreds of miles away (MacQueen, 1986). Integration of education and nursing services allows a child with cystic fibrosis or developmental handicaps to receive timely evaluation, speedy entry into the best educational placement, and monitoring of the child's growth and development as they are affected by schooling and health care. The ventilator-dependent child who is homebound receives intervention services there because of the effective working relationships between health and education services at the local and regional levels. Family advocates in Iowa assist families to find services, work with health payers to improve benefits, and help parents learn to nurture their children (Iowa).

La Rabida Hospital in Chicago, a major childhood chronic illness inpatient facility, offers a refreshing example of comprehensive care. Discharge planning begins on the day of admission, even for children whose hospitalizations may last for months. Families play a central role in this planning, and the staff's comprehensive view of the process includes evaluation of the home's physical environment; preparation of equipment for the home and provision for its maintenance; teaching parents and other family members about the child's care; organization of community-based treatment services; and plans for respite care, educational programs, and social services. The program allows for gradually longer periods of time of home trial, when families try out the experience of having their child at home.

Some school districts provide a combination of special and regular classrooms in the same school setting, where, however, extensive nursing and other health services are more readily available than in other school buildings. One program is the Neil School in Chicago, a public school that serves 200 handicapped youngsters in the special education section of the facility and 200 able-bodied children with 22 handicapped children in the other. The school employs four nurses and several other therapists who perform a variety of health procedures, allowing the children to stay in classes appropriate to their educational level.

New York Hospital's Regional Hemophilia Center organizes a comprehensive array of services for children with hemophilia and their families. Hemophilia is one of the success stories in home care for youngsters. Development of blood products that can be administered at home, avoiding hospitalization or emergency room treatment, has revolutionized the ways children and adults with hemophilia care for their illness (Smith & Levine, 1984). The Regional Hemophilia Center has been a leader in this revolution. In the past, children with severe hemophilia had one to three hospitalizations per month to treat bleeding in their joints. Now, quicker and cheaper care is provided by home infusion. Yet hemophilia, like most other serious long-term illnesses, creates special tasks for the child and family. Blood replacement factors and the equipment to administer them are costly, the disease and its treatments may have complications that require further monitoring and treatment, and the additional stress may cause mental health problems. Many children and adults with hemophilia are HIV-positive because of contamination during the early 1980s of replacement factors with the AIDS virus. The New York Hospital program, aiming to maximize the likelihood that children will be at home rather than in the hospital, addresses medical, educational, and social services, rather than limiting its attention to monitoring the bleeding status of children with hemophilia.

In Maryland, an independent agency provides care coordination for families, especially those whose children have severe long-term illnesses that require attention from a large number of health specialists and extensive home nursing and other therapies. The team of nurse-coordinators, family resource and education planners, medical personnel, and financial specialists at the Coordinating Center for Home and Community Care assures that families receive the supports they need to make home care successful.

These programs are distinguished by recognition that families provide the majority of care for their own children when the conditions are severe or require major technologies in the home. That these programs alone cannot meet all of the needs of families is documented by the many continuing concerns articulated by parents in this study who receive services from these exemplary programs. The programs have successfully strengthened families' abilities through comprehensive and coordinated approaches to delivering services. These model programs exemplify elements of the most effective care for children and families. If tied into a broader system emphasizing comprehensiveness, continuity, and coordination, these programs can be the nucleus of services that work.

SUMMARY

Services currently available to families are often fragmented, poorly coordinated, and limited in their scope, such that many family needs go unmet. Many children lack access to programs that integrate the four main systems of care: community-based home health and nursing care, hospitals, schools, and other community services. Organized systems are the exception rather than the rule. Parents face an uphill battle in their attempt to have a role in key decisions for their child and in directing the child's program. The current organizational system favors services provided at the centralized hospital level, but the very nature of home-based care calls for complex services to be provided at home. Important experiments have begun to integrate home and hospital services in the continuum of care, but the demonstration must be extended to a much larger segment of the population.

Optimally, the child should be in a school setting that best responds to his or her intellectual and social abilities, with as little interference from the child's illness as possible. Parents need help in assessing the educational needs and capacities of their child. Schools require assistance in understanding the implications of the student's illness for educational attainment and classroom participation so that they can provide barrier-free access to the correct special *or* regular classrooms. Medication policies and means for integrating special equipment, treatments, and personnel should all be in place.

To nurture their children, families require not only medical and surgical services but also nursing care, education about illness and its treatment, support to obtain the best educational placement for their child, mental health counseling, and social services especially to help finance care and to access community resources and agencies. Furthermore, services must be continuous, comprehensive, and coordinated. In the next chapter we turn to the exploration of these benchmarks of quality of care.

4

Quality of Home Care

Chrissy Ericksen has always needed the support of a ventilator to help her breathe. As a premature newborn weighing only 18 ounces (700 grams) at birth, she developed bronchopulmonary dysplasia and spent the first 18 months of her life in the hospital. Now three years old, having been home for a year and a half, Chrissy is cared for by home care nurses 20 hours each day. With the support of her pulmonary specialist at the children's hospital, she is beginning to be weaned from the ventilator. She also receives physical therapy and speech therapy from the local early intervention program. A respiratory therapist checks in every month to provide preventive maintenance to the equipment. Chrissy's father is a self-employed gas station owner and mechanic; her mother would rather stay home with Chrissy but remains in her job as office manager at the school superintendent's office in order to keep the family's group health insurance.

The Ericksens worked closely with the home care nursing agency in selecting nurses to care for Chrissy. They made it a point to interview all nurses before allowing them into their home. They refused to accept nurses who were unfamiliar with Chrissy's equipment, who did not understand children and their development, or with whom they were uncomfortable. They insisted that nurses who were otherwise acceptable but lacked knowledge of the equipment receive special in-service training at the specialty care hospital 40 miles from their home.

At first, the supervisor at the home care agency was annoyed that the Ericksens were so demanding. "What do they expect?" she often wondered. But as time passed, the supervisor saw that the Ericksens had few complaints about nursing care and that the nurses assigned to work with Chrissy enjoyed their jobs, rarely called in sick, never had car problems that kept them from work, and almost never quit.

Chrissy crawls and is beginning to walk. The limitations on her explorations because of her tether to the ventilator and her difficulty in communicating have made her so frustrated that she has frequent temper tantrums. The tantrums are especially frightening to her parents and the nurses because, in addition to kicking and beating the floor, she holds her breath or pulls out her tracheostomy tube. At the insistence of the Ericksens, the home-care nurses, the speech therapist, the general pediatrician in their community who follows Chrissy, and the Ericksens themselves are working together to decrease the frequency of the tantrums and to encourage Chrissy's language development in order to lessen her frustration.

The Ericksens provide a good example of how home care can be made to work well and how quality care can be provided with the vigilance and assertiveness of parents working in partnership with professionals. The Ericksens have made their situation work by demanding quality services, by coordinating care for their child, and by collaborating *with* the nurses on whom they are so dependent. Working in their favor are their management skills developed at their workplaces and their suburban community that has an ample cadre of health professionals so that they can be selective about the nurses who will care for their daughter.

Few families enjoy home care of the quality experienced by the Ericksens. Families usually begin home care without the management skills that the Ericksens bring to the experience. Few are able to coordinate care without special assistance, especially when their children are first at home. And few families live in communities with an abundance of health care resources; refusing to accept a nurse for home care is not an option for families where there are few nurses in the community.

Quality services are essential for home care to be safe and effective in meeting the needs of children and families. Quality home care will increase children's chances of achieving their maximal potential. Furthermore, access to quality services—competent nurses, adequate respite care, supportive physicians, and appropriate therapies—enhances the ability of families to stick with the rigors of home care.

ASSESSING THE QUALITY OF HOME CARE

How can quality of home care be assessed and assured? What mechanisms improve quality? Comments and observations from the site visits indicate that many families as well as physicians and case managers are dissatisfied with the quality of home care, especially with home-care nursing. This problem surfaced in virtually all communities visited, urban and rural, North and South; and examples of inadequate care were disturbingly numerous. Many people providing home care are effective and committed, yet the variability in standards, monitoring of services, and training of providers is enormous.

Overall, attention to improving the quality of home care has been minimal.

Families must select from a vast array of services as they begin home care—home health agencies, equipment vendors, medical supply companies, community physicians, and pharmacies, to name a few. Choosing among the services and determining their quality can be formidable tasks. Families identify many problems relating to quality of care: quality of home-care service providers, family management of home-care services, and inadequate coordination of services. An understanding of the elements of quality care provides a structure from which to discuss strategies to improve the quality of home care for children with special health care needs.

The quality of care that a child receives at home or elsewhere is determined both by the knowledge of the practitioner and by the skill with which he or she delivers the care. Knowledge of procedures is fairly straightforward: Either the nurse knows how to change a tracheostomy tube or does not. But skillful delivery involves more than changing the tube properly. It involves recognizing the emotional concerns and fears of the child and parents and addressing them appropriately. Knowledge of the technical aspects of a procedure is necessary but not sufficient. Technical skills must be complemented by an understanding of how to work with a child and family to carry out the procedure—the interpersonal or affective aspects of care.

Providing technical care and procedures in the home is only one aspect of quality. How the care systems respond to the child's and family's needs is equally important. Are the nursing services readily and consistently available? Is the child enrolled in school? Do the nurses communicate with the teachers at school about the changing needs of the child? These questions reflect the responsiveness of the system of care to the broader development of the child and the integration of the family into the community.

Donabedian (1980) described two major areas for the evaluation of quality of health care—personal care and the system of care. Quality of personal care includes three elements: the technical or procedural care, interpersonal issues in providing care, and the amenities with which care is provided. The quality of the system of care is a function also of three factors: continuity, access, and coordination. These areas correspond with the major concerns voiced by families and program staff and the problems that were observed during the site visits.

The quality of technical or procedural care focuses on the mechanisms of providing care. The Ericksens addressed their concerns about the quality of technical care when they insisted that nurses unfamiliar with the equipment used by their daughter receive special training from the specialty center. Technical care encompasses more than management of high-tech equipment such as ventilators, tracheostomy tubes, and gastrostomy tubes. It also includes procedures for monitoring the positive and negative effects of medications, changing dressings by nurses, carrying out specific muscle exercises by physical therapists, and evaluating fevers through such activities as examining ears for infections and listening to a congested chest through a stethoscope.

The issue of interpersonal care focuses on how providers relate with families. The Ericksens refused to allow nurses with whom they were uncomfortable to care for Chrissy. They believed that interpersonal problems that would hinder the development of a good working relationship were more likely to arise if the initial interview with the nurse went poorly. Other families and program staff at the site visits noted with great frequency the interpersonal problems with home-care providers, mostly nurses since they most often provide care.

The amenities of personal care are important to the lives of families who have frequent contact with health care providers. On-time appointments, comfortable and welcoming waiting rooms, convenient and inexpensive parking, and on-site child-care services for siblings are among the many amenities that the personal care system can offer. For families whose children are at home, amenities also encompass special issues about the home environment such as alarms, noise levels, or air conditioning.

A central issue in the continuity of the system of care is whether a person is able to see the same health care providers on an ongoing basis. For families with children with long-term health conditions, this feature of quality care takes on special meaning. Seeing the same provider means not having to repeat at each visit the child's lengthy medical history in less than one minute; an ongoing provider remembers the child's background and has access to records that will document his or her history, making the recitation superfluous. Seeing the same provider also means that tests will not be repeated unnecessarily, avoiding extra expense for the family and discomfort for the child. For those in home care, continuity of home-care providers, such as the stable group of nurses who take care of Chrissy Ericksen, offers parents assurance that their child is in competent hands and that therapy is continuing as prescribed.

Access to the system of care considers such issues as whether services are available in the community, whether families can get to the services, and whether financial requirements bar families from getting services. For families whose children receive home care, availability of services alone does not assure access. Transportation problems, language barriers for parents who do not speak fluent English, and financial barriers because of the high cost of some services effectively block access even when services are available.

Coordination of care requires that the multiple providers of care from the various systems that serve the child and family work in concert to achieve optimal results for all. Coordination requires that someone have responsibility for assuring that all providers exchange pertinent information. For Chrissy Ericksen, the care coordinators are her parents, but other children may lack care coordinators. The importance of coordination for assuring quality care for children with complex medical conditions was discussed in Chapter 3.

PERSONAL CARE

Technical and Interpersonal Care

How good are the technical care and the interpersonal skills of health care providers for children with severe long-term illnesses and their families? Nurses provide much home care, and nursing's crucial importance in this field merits special attention. However, the quality of other home care providers—physical therapists, respiratory therapists, equipment technicians—is also critical.

Nurses caring for children at home typically have greater responsibilities than do nurses in hospitals and require more sophisticated knowledge. Home care nurses work alone. They must assess subtle changes in the child's condition that may indicate the need for hospitalization, changes in medical treatments, or help from physicians or other health providers. Yet many home-care nurses have little training in inpatient pediatrics or the home care of children (VNS). Many have backgrounds in the home care of the elderly or care of in-hospital patients that leave them ill-prepared to work with severely ill children and their families at home. Moreover, few nurses have experience with the sophisticated equipment used at home by technology-dependent children.

A nurse working in a home setting has much less supervision and available advice and consultation than does a nurse on a hospital inpatient unit. Nurses in home care work more independently, almost as solo practitioners. They can contact fellow nurses or other health consultants by phone, but they lack the informal quick advice and camaraderie that comes from fellow practitioners working side by side every day in a hospital or office setting. Nurses in offices and hospitals can ask colleagues to help evaluate a child or family; in homes, they are mainly on their own (Aday, Aitken, & Wegener, 1988).

Many home-care agencies have had the demands of an expanding pediatric population thrust on them by hospitals, third-party payers, and governmental agencies. Yet many agencies are too poorly staffed with appropriately trained providers to offer quality services; they have too few providers who understand the needs of children in home care and the requirements of the technology. Although the administrative staff of agencies recognize these problems, they lack the resources and support to improve training to keep pace with referrals.

These limitations were underscored by Feinberg (1985). "The unique technical requirements of this pediatric population are often not understood by an industry that is oriented to adults. Parents report episodes of nurses who arrive to care for their ventilator dependent children who have never seen a ventilator [and] suppliers who bring incorrect supplies" (p. 41). Similarly, Thorp (1987) observed equipment-related problems, especially monitor malfunctions, unreliable nursing coverage, last-minute cancellations, and incompetence. One mother said, "People think 24-hour nursing is easy street. You have problems all the way" (p. 136).

Although most nurses practice responsibly, some nurses are negligent in carrying out their duties. Home-care coordinators at one site related their concern about the care afforded several children. In spite of having professional nursing care 20 hours a day, an 8-year-old girl with a brain tumor and tracheostomy living at the Maryland shore had dressings that had not been changed in 13 days. A 13-month-old boy in Washington, DC, on a ventilator because of premature birth, has bronchopulmonary dysplasia. He has 24-hour nursing coverage because his mother, now four months pregnant, goes into labor when she gets out of bed. The night nurse, however, leaves before her replacement arrives. Care coordinators said that these instances of neglect typify the difficulty of obtaining adequate nursing services in many locales, both urban and rural (Maryland).

Even when nurses carry out the technical requirements of providing home care for children responsibly, troubling interpersonal issues arise. With daily exposure to the home, some nurses become over-involved with the family, discipline the children in their care or the siblings, or disagree with the family about how to perform procedures. On the other hand, the daily exposure leads some families to expect home-care nurses to reveal their personal lives, undermining a strictly professional relationship. In some instances, nurses have openly disapproved of a parent's life-style (for instance, a mother living with her boyfriend). On one site visit, a nurse related the problem of distinguishing between parents' punishment by spankings, of which she did not approve, and child abuse, which she is required to report by law. Not surprisingly, most nurses report that they are uncomfortable dealing with these types of family issues (Illinois).

Problems with interpersonal care extend to thoughtless treatment by home-care workers. The mother of David, an 18-year-old boy with severe cerebral palsy, has cared for him without nursing assistance since his birth. Shift nursing care recently became necessary when David became ventilator-dependent and bedridden after an asphyxiation episode. The night nurse, a large, brusque woman, has a boyfriend who comes to the house or calls late in the evening. The mother's requests that this behavior stop have been ignored by the nurse and the agency. Several of the day nurses are kind and thoughtful, but they are so poorly trained in using the equipment that David's mother is afraid to leave him in their care. She fears that nursing services will be discontinued if she insists on personnel changes (Maryland).

Given the difficulty of finding nurses who are well trained in the home care of children, one mother told us that she is willing to accept nurses with appropriate interpersonal skills even if their technical training is insufficient. "The right personality and high self-confidence are the most important qualities of a good nurse." Although she prefers to hire nurses with pediatric backgrounds, the mother waives this requirement if the personality traits seem to be a good match. She believes that training nurses to carry out procedures correctly is easier than teaching them how to relate to the family (Personal communication, Kaileigh Mulligan Program family interview, 1988).

Not all responsibility for inadequate care falls on the shoulders of professionals. In some instances, families create situations that undermine opportunities for positive interpersonal relations. One family in Maryland would not permit nurses to communicate at shift changes, making it nearly impossible for the new nurse coming on to know important changes in the child that had occurred during the previous shift. In another situation, the father purposely walked naked through the house to the irritation of the home-care nurses. These examples illustrate some of the ways in which families themselves undermine the ability of caregivers to establish the interpersonal relationships needed for care of the highest quality.

In addition to the problems with home-care nursing services, families frequently experience problems with equipment dealers and service representatives. Care coordinators in Illinois told of ventilators being shipped to the family by package delivery services. The families were then expected to unpack, install, and maintain the equipment themselves. In another instance, parents described an equipment service technician who was so inept that they would no longer permit him to enter the house. In frustration, the father taught himself how to maintain and repair his son's ventilator (Illinois).

Physicians have a limited role in home care. When the child is in the hospital, the physician is a major player on the care team and in planning for discharge. But when the child goes home, the hospital-based physician becomes less central to the child's daily care. This change in emphasis is borne out by families, who had little to say about the physician's role in home care or the quality of services they provide.

The few physicians who do remain involved in home care voiced concerns about the quality of care provided by peers and colleagues. Physicians' worries about increased liability and fear of litigation affect their willingness to support home care for technology-dependent children. Some physicians fear that the home is less safe than the hospital and that they may therefore face a lawsuit for discharging a stable but medically complex child to home. Doctors worry also about their liability when they approve a home nursing care plan without knowing the skill level of the home-care nurses or if the nurses are up-to-date with the technology needed by the child (Illinois). A pediatrician in the Midwest expressed the strong belief that to maintain quality care the community pediatrician must remain closely involved with the family and avoid extra referrals. He feels that, as the number of referrals increases, the community physician becomes less involved in the child's care and may lose track of the child's progress or setbacks. In his judgment, a single person should oversee medical care for a chronically ill child to assure "consistency of commitment." This pediatrician also believes that families should be responsible for directing the home care of their children, even if mistakes are made and the child suffers a small setback. In this way, the family has an opportunity to learn and grow (Iowa).

The erosion of the quality of care when community-based physicians disassociate themselves from a child receiving care at home was observed by an Illinois pediatrician. He noted that few ventilator-dependent children have a primary-care physician or receive continuing follow-up to reassess their tertiary care needs. More typically, the main task of the attending physician from the medical center, who may rarely see the child after discharge, is to reorder the home-care services. Lack of acquaintance with the specifics of the home situation on the part of physicians may mean that they reorder home nursing care without reassessing the child and family situation. Ongoing services, therefore, may not reflect the changing needs of the family and may be inappropriate for the child's condition (Illinois). Better care at the community level would help make these services more reflective of the needs of both child and family.

Amenities

The amenities of care when a child is home reflect the intrusiveness of the child's technological support, the need for regular professional caregivers, and the underlying home environment. Few families voice complaints about the amenities of home care. Indeed, most families seem so delighted with the major benefit of home care—that the child is home in the nurturing environment of the family and that regular, costly, time-consuming trips to the hospital are no longer needed—that amenities are overlooked.

Homes that accommodate severely ill children run the gamut from a four-bedroom suburban home in the Midwest, to an immaculately kept apartment in a housing project in the Bronx, New York, to a rundown cottage in northern Florida, heated on cold days with a kerosene space heater. Nevertheless, whatever the environment, the parents in this study wanted their children at home. Technological invasions of the home—blaring televisions to placate a child, whirring ventilators creating low-level background noise, alarms from malfunctioning equipment—are necessary for a child's care but impair the living situation for the entire family. There is often no alternative to accepting these intrusions with their potential negative impact on the family.

By far the most significant effect on life styles is the regular presence of professional caregivers in the home. Just as nurses are uncomfortable dealing with personal issues of home life, so too are families disrupted by the outsiders. Additional caretakers in the home create a loss of privacy and a loss of control of the family's life. Concerns of family members include the sharing of bathroom facilities, the worry of others overhearing normal family arguments or seeing them discipline their children, and the difficulties of maintaining normal intimate relationships in what are now more public surroundings. Different standards of personal dress or even of housecleaning may be needed when there is a continuing flow of strangers into the home (La Rabida).

Even with home care, families continue to have frequent contact with the health care system outside the home. Regular outpatient visits, unexpected trips to the emergency room, and hospitalizations continue. In general, few amenities are offered to families who receive these services. Sitting in waiting rooms with uncomfortable chairs, long waits when providers run behind schedule, or hospital rooms that are inadequately cleaned are frequent reminders to families of missing amenities. When asked the hypothetical question of what she would do if she had the funds to improve the care her son receives, one mother laughed and replied, "Look around you. I would fix up this place." She pointed to examination rooms that were separated by curtains, offering almost no privacy, equipment that was old and outdated, and offices with shabby furnishings (Einstein).

SYSTEM OF CARE

Continuity

Continuity of care is a major determinant of quality. Families lose confidence in a care system whose face constantly changes or whose staff knows little about the history of the child. Unfortunately, the nursing agencies providing most home care for children with severe medical conditions suffer from several problems that undermine continuity. Most home nursing staff have intense, demanding jobs and large workloads. The nature of the nurses' jobs often leads to isolation and emotional stress brought on by the difficult or unfortunate family situations. And because they work in isolation, the nurses lack emotional support from their own colleagues. The heavy demands of their work lead to staff burnout, with high turnover of nurses and little continuity of care.

Families discussing the nursing care of their children who are ventilator-dependent often say that the first cadre of nurses is well prepared to provide care, having often been trained by the tertiary-care hospital in planning for home discharge. Unfortunately, as these nurses resign, their replacements may be untrained for the tasks at hand (La Rabida). To compensate, many families strengthen their own skills in the use of technological devices at home and in the complex nursing care of their child. Nevertheless, the diminishing quality and preparation of nursing personnel threaten families' sense of confidence that the system works for them. Certainly, as children's health status improves, families will likely need less sophisticated nursing care over time; but changes should come through careful planning rather than through staff burnout and turnover.

Continuous physician care is essential for quality care for children with complicated medical histories. Most families that we met experienced continuity of physicians, at least for specialty care, but this observation is in part biased by the route through which we found families: through programs that were, in many cases, run by physicians and well staffed with a stable group of doctors.

Other families relate the problem of bouncing from physician to physician either by their own choice because of dissatisfaction with providers (Iowa) or because of the organization of the clinics where they receive care. Such discontinuity of care is costly in a number of ways. Economic costs are high as physicians retest children to confirm for themselves previously established results. In effect, each visit is a lengthy "first" visit. Costs for family time are also considerable. The cost of annoyance to the family in frequent recitations of the child's medical history cannot be discounted. Some advocacy groups recommend that parents maintain a one-page summary of the child's medical history to obviate a tedious, time-consuming, and often incomplete recitation for each new provider. Finally, the cost in terms of medical outcome of discontinuous care is high. Children who lack an ongoing medical care provider suffer from having no long-term plan to promote their medical well-being.

Access and Choice

Many families face barriers to services that support home care. Potential
barriers to access are lack of funding for the service or the lack of availability
of the service in the community in a culturally appropriate fashion. Chapter 6
looks at funding issues. We focus here on the questions of availability and
cultural appropriateness.

The broad range of services that families need—medical, social, psychological, recreational, and educational—is more available in urban areas, albeit
with various limitations, than in rural communities where services are limited.
One family living in rural Florida described the joy of bringing home their 17-
month-old son and the difficulty of finding services for him. They realized
that, if they could not find local services, they would have to uproot the family
and move. They wrote ungrammatically but eloquently, ''With all the stress
we had, because we live so far from everything this was and still is an issue, an
issue that I to this day find so MADDENING. Here our son has tryed so hard
to come home. He has been through more than my Husband and I put together
and where we live is an issue. . . . Now we would do anything for our son
and go anywhere for him, but we wanted to settle down for a while, get him
settled and use to his surroundings. So we are fighting for his Upcoming
Education. If we loose then the house goes We guess'' (Personal communication, Florida family, 1990).

Availability is also curtailed, in both urban and rural communities, when
services are offered by only one provider. In most communities, only one
specialty group (for example, one hemophilia or arthritis treatment program)
exists. The lack of choice limits families' opportunities to select providers
whom they prefer. Similarly, families living on the rural Maryland shore may
have only one choice for a home-care nursing provider; if this agency proves
to be unacceptable, the family has no alternative. Freedom of choice is limited
when families have few options.

For children at home with severe medical conditions, access to physicians,
especially community-based primary care providers, is deficient for several
reasons. Many families report that they are unable to obtain care from community pediatricians for their children. In some instances, parents do not trust
these physicians to have sufficient expertise in the care of their children's
problems and so seek alternate sources for medical care. Some parents report,
further, that community physicians are uncomfortable with their ability to
care for such complex children and will instead refer the youngsters to specialists for care. Community-based pediatricians are poorly compensated by insurance for the extra time for counseling, coordinating care, and other supportive activities that are essential to the care of a child with a complex medical

condition; the economics of running a practice make it nearly impossible for these physicians to care for such complex children. Finally, many community-based physicians refuse Medicaid patients, thereby excluding many children with complex medical conditions. One foster mother from the suburbs of Chicago described the unwillingness of her own child's pediatrician to provide care to her foster son, who was Medicaid-eligible (La Rabida).

Many other needed services are unavailable. Respite care, day care, and mainstream recreational opportunities, such as Boy Scouts or swimming classes, which accept children with complex medical conditions, are examples of programs that are rarely found in communities, either urban or rural. These limitations place tremendous pressures on families either to plan special outings, to provide services themselves, or to do without.

Cultural differences create obstacles to access to services. Language barriers making communication difficult are the most common examples of cultural differences undermining availability. Other cultural issues impair the ability of mothers to make use of those services that are available. Some cultures place men (for example, husbands or boyfriends) in strongly dominant and domineering roles. One case manager described the importance of meeting the household's dominant male in order to enlist his cooperation and support for treatments; without the support of the man of the house, the case manager knew that the mother would not follow through with treatment plans (Personal communication, Children's Medical Services, Florida, 1989).

Coordination

Specific services provided to a child and family may be of high quality, but the total package may be inadequate because of a lack of coordination. Chapter 3 described the importance of coordination for families, and others have documented the multiple disciplines and many service providers in the care of children with complex long-term illnesses (Ireys, 1981; Klerman, 1985). Lack of coordination of these services leads to conflicts and competing priorities among services, duplication of some activities, and lack of access to still others. Coordination is a central element of quality care.

The barriers to coordinating care are extensive. Providers from disparate disciplines, based at great geographic distances, have little contact with each other, making coordination of effort awkward at best. Professionals are rarely compensated for coordination efforts, so finding time to allocate for this activity is difficult. Reluctance to share information among professionals and to risk violating client confidentiality creates additional obstacles. Finally, professionals from different disciplines—medicine, education, nursing, psychology and others—often have difficulty working together as a team.

Hospital discharge is a transitional time when coordination is especially critical. Without appropriate planning, hospital discharge is postponed. A child in New York with a tracheostomy who required full-time nursing care was about to be discharged to the custody of her grandmother who worked full-time outside the home (COPE). Such a home-care situation can work well if adequate home nursing services are arranged; but, in this case, the hospital discharge planners had neglected to coordinate with the grandmother. They had assumed that she was available for round-the-clock daily care and had not arranged nursing coverage. In another instance, a grandmother caring for a child with severe developmental delay agreed to a package of specialized therapies for the grandchild, believing that her agreement was necessary for the child's release from the hospital. Shortly after the child went home, the grandmother discontinued many of the home therapies (COPE). Poor cooperation between hospital-based discharge planners and home caregivers undermines the quality of home care. Furthermore, poor communication by discharge planners can lead also to extra, unnecessary services. A developmentally delayed child was discharged from a rehabilitation hospital in the Northeast with home nursing provided by the hospital's home health agency. Physical and occupational therapy was requested from the Visiting Nurse Association, but lack of adequate communication led to the VNA's provision of home nursing services, duplicating the hospital's nursing services (Personal communication, Boston VNA, 1987).

Coordination *within* the medical care system when a child is at home is also fraught with difficulties, partly because of poor communication between specialty providers and primary care physicians who are involved with the child's treatment. The child with Goldenhar's syndrome, described earlier in this text, has multiple health providers: a general pediatrician; pulmonary specialists; ear, nose, and throat specialists; surgeons; speech therapists; and cardiologists, among others. When the child's mother receives conflicting advice, such as about the use of a neck collar that will interfere with the child's tracheostomy tube, she laboriously consults with others but finally uses her professional skills to decide the best course for her son.

Problems of coordination within the medical care system alone are difficult enough to resolve. When problems arise among multiple disciplines, difficulties can grow exponentially. To resolve conflicting advice from the home-care physical therapist and the child's pediatrician, a mother called the pediatrician during the therapist's visit to force a discussion of the issues (VNS). Other problems are less amenable to easy resolution. The parents of a ventilator-dependent girl, with the support of the pediatrician, wanted her to attend school with her peers, but neither the school nor Medicaid was willing to fund the private-duty nursing care necessary for her to attend safely. Extensive litigation was required before this conflict was resolved (*Detsel v. Sullivan*, 1990). While coordination alone may not have solved the latter problem, the first issue, a conflict between the physical therapist and pediatrician, would have been easily negotiated with the assistance of a care coordinator.

Coordination of services and machines from medical equipment companies is another responsibility of families. Unfortunately, families often do not learn of unsafe equipment or supplies because they themselves are outside the communication network. Respiratory therapists in a hospital will usually hear of problems with specific pieces of equipment; the family, more isolated, may go for a long period of time unaware that their machinery is defective or unsafe. Lack of coordination between specialty services and the home again extends the family's burdens (Illinois).

Effective care coordination is essential to assuring quality of care. The tasks involved in coordination of a child's care and the people responsible for coordination change as the youngster progresses through the health care system from the hospital to the discharge-planning phase to home. In the hospital, the coordinator is often the attending physician or the nurses most directly responsible for the child's care. As hospital discharge is anticipated, discharge planners, usually nurses or social workers employed by hospitals, assume responsibility for planning the transition from hospital to home. But once the child is home, responsibility for care coordination is less clear. While most families feel that they are responsible for care coordination, most need help in learning to negotiate the community service system.

That effective coordination can develop is demonstrated by the several programs previously described: Pediatric Home Care; the multidisciplinary hemophilia team at New York Hospital; Project REACH; the Maryland Coordinating Center. Adequate coordination requires a means of easy communication and occasional meetings. As members of the provider team change, new members need to be fully introduced to the family and explicitly trained in the specific issues for this child and family. But through all the transitions, the family remains in charge as the ultimate coordinator of care.

Family members must be central members of the child's care team. They must approve plans developed by the team and be involved in all key decisions. The independence with which professionals such as nurses function in the home calls for new alliances: the family as fellow observer and as senior partner in the monitoring and formulation of plans. The notion of family involvement applies to other types of health care provision; but in the context of home care it takes on an even more compelling importance. The isolation felt by families, by nurses, and by other health professionals can be mitigated by the formation of a collaboration that shares the many tasks of observation, monitoring, direct care, and training and education.

IMPROVING THE QUALITY OF HOME CARE

How can the quality of home care be improved? Donabedian (1980) described a framework for assessing quality with three elements: the structure, process, and outcome of care. Simply put, structure includes the organization and elements of the system of care; process considers the way in which care is provided; and outcome looks at the effects on the patient, family, or society.

Outcomes of care, such as the health or functioning of the child and family, are the ultimate indicators of home-care quality and as such may be viewed as more important than the structure of services or the process of care (Donabedian, 1989). It is hoped that care provided well (with high quality in the structure and process of care) will maximize the likelihood of positive outcomes, yet measurement of outcomes can be quite difficult, especially for children whose conditions are chronic and will not be cured. Nevertheless, intermediate outcome goals can apply to children with long-term severe illnesses and to their families, and recent work to measure a child's health in terms of resilience, psychological status, adaptability, or physical functioning provide methods to assess outcomes (Stein & Jessop, 1990; Tarlov et al., 1989)

Structure

The structure of services considers such issues as numbers and types of personnel employed; the qualifications of nurses and other staff; the training, supervision, and monitoring of staff; and the organization of programs, for example, whether for-profit or not-for-profit, centralized or decentralized, small or large size. Some state and community supervisory agencies argue that minimum standards must be developed for the programs that provide home care. They contend that standards will improve the quality of home care programs that currently employ nurses with limited pediatric skills and will eliminate the problem of nurses who lack the technical skills for the job. These agencies recommend specification of the level of training necessary for a home health worker and the development of procedures to assess and assure that care at home is of high caliber. Some have recommended the certification of providers of professional home-care services in addition to the licensure of home-care agencies; this strategy has been used in Minnesota (Ginsburg, 1986). Others have a policy of contracting only with home-care agencies that have established affiliations with other providers of quality care (Applebaum & Christianson, 1988).

Requiring home-care agencies to meet explicit standards of personnel training, supervision, and experience is another method that has been used to improve the quality of home-care. The Blue Cross/Blue Shield program in Maryland hopes to improve the quality of home-care agencies by offering financial incentives to agencies that meet the established standards. Agencies meeting such standards receive provisional acceptance as a registered provider for one year. The Blue Cross/Blue Shield program then monitors the agency's work for the year, and if no problems arise in that time, the agency becomes a regular registered provider (Maryland). Some case managers have performed a similar role by authorizing services for elderly clients from only those agencies that meet staff training and supervision requirements (Applebaum & Christianson, 1988).

Will setting standards and qualifications for home-care agencies and providers improve the quality of home care? Will the Maryland Blue Cross/Blue Shield program to monitor agency standards improve the quality of services provided? How applicable are standards to the home care setting where lay caregivers such as parents, extended family, and neighbors are expected to provide the majority of care?

The issue of standards and agency accreditation is complex; nevertheless, it seems clear that the professionals involved with families in home care must meet basic standards of professional accreditation and licensure, that staff must demonstrate special expertise in the area of children's care, and that all providers must have explicit training in areas related to the specific child in home-care. These elements are necessary but insufficient to assure quality in home care. While able to increase the likelihood that home-care nurses are technically competent, standards will not address the problems that families experience with interpersonal care. When placed in a broader context of a system of home care, standards will help resolve some of the problems that families report.

Questions about standards and qualifications of home-care service providers apply also to coordinators. Professional care coordinators come from a variety of backgrounds, such as nursing, education, social work, counseling, and the clergy. This variety reflects the range of tasks assigned to coordinators: direct care; financial counseling; coordination among medical providers; teaching about the child's care needs; emotional support; coordination among the medical, education, and home nursing systems; help in finding services for the child; and teaching families to provide care coordination on their own. Five program directors around the country described with remarkable similarity the personality characteristics of care coordinators: persistent, outgoing, good sense of humor, creative, flexible, assertive, and having good communication skills. Yet few standards for training and qualifications of care coordinators exist, making assessment difficult.

Reimbursement issues, both the level of payment to home care agencies and the determination of reimbursable services, greatly influence the quality of home care (Applebaum & Christianson, 1988). Payment to home-care agency providers is sometimes reputedly too low to hire quality staff. Low reimbursement leads to low wage scales. This strategy undermines the quality of home care by attracting less able employees and by encouraging greater employee turnover. Furthermore, it discourages employee training because of the accompanying costs and the limited benefit to the agency when employees' tenure is short. Increased reimbursement for home-care services would help to alleviate these problems.

Third-party payers' policies about reimbursable services sometimes discourage the provision of needed home-care services. For instance, the refusal of insurers to reimburse for case management or for care conferences limits the provision of these services. Without these services, children's access to care may suffer and coordination will be more difficult. Other financing strategies to improve quality have been observed. Case managers for elderly clients had the impression that cost sharing (applied to only upper income clients) increased clients' willingness to report problems with the quality of care (Applebaum & Christianson, 1988).

Process

The process of care describes the mechanisms by which care is provided: how nurses use their time, how equipment is employed to monitor or treat a health condition, what medications a child is given, or what school services a child receives at home. Although the process of care is not always related to outcomes, the appropriate process of care is more likely to improve a child's health status.

Parents and their children, especially children who are older, are often in the best position to evaluate the quality of the care process, especially for home care where there is little staff supervision. Parents are often able to assess the quality of technical care; and they are often the only people who are able to evaluate the quality of interpersonal care (Davies & Ware, 1988).

Improving the quality of the process of care is most often accomplished by developing guidelines for care and including these guidelines in training. Guidelines for home care must reflect the special circumstances of the home environment and the unique needs of children. Although some investigators contend that guidelines for care that is transferred from the hospital to the home (e.g., the care of a ventilator dependent child) should reflect hospital-based protocols (Kane, 1991), the circumstances of the home require additional considerations. Special characteristics of children—their evolving development and physical growth—must be considered in establishing standards of care. Thus, existing protocols for hospital care can serve as a starting point for developing new guidelines for home care. Storage of medications, cleaning and maintenance of equipment, and preparation of special diets are all examples that may need modification in their transfer from the hospital to the home.

Continuity of home-care staff helps to improve the quality of the process of care. Several programs have attempted to improve the continuity of care by reducing turnover of nursing staff. The staff of Pediatric Home Care in New York meets weekly to discuss each child currently enrolled in the program, partly to meet concerns about nurses' isolation and lack of peer education and support. These sessions provide an opportunity for regular training and patient care supervision. If a family faces special problems, the staff member working most closely with the family presents the situation to colleagues and seeks advice. In addition, the team of a pediatrician and pediatric nurse practitioner meets periodically to discuss joint cases. In a similar fashion, Florida's Project REACH arranged weekly meetings at a central location for the community-based nurses who coordinated the home care for severely ill children. Meeting topics included issues affecting specific families, updates on clinical care of specific illnesses, and principles of care coordination. Access to discussion with colleagues provides support for staff in emotionally draining roles, diminishes isolation, reduces staff turnover by alleviating burnout, and adds to staff knowledge; the quality of care provided by the group as a whole improves.

Several strategies can improve the quality of the care process. Written lists that specify a home care provider's duties, prominently posted in the home and shared with providers and agencies, can improve quality by making expectations explicit to all. Where this method has been used (mainly in home care of elderly patients), family caregivers became more aware of the extent of the services that home-care providers were expected to offer (Applebaum & Christianson, 1988).

Case managers can improve the process of care by using several simple techniques that were described by Applebaum and Christianson (1988). Timing home visits to coincide with home-care service providers allows case managers to observe the home visit and assess the quality of care. Phone calls to the home, scheduled during a home-care visit, help case managers document late visits or no-shows. Case managers can then share with each other the performance of particular providers or agencies to identify patterns of high and poor quality. Agencies unable to improve quality and providers whose performance remain substandard receive fewer referrals by the case managers.

Staff of New England SERVE (1989) developed guidelines for families (or providers) to help them assess services offered by care providers and agencies.

These guidelines focus mainly on the process of care offered by personal health services, health care providers and teams, health care agencies, state health departments, and community-based programs. The SERVE guidelines provide insight into policies and procedures that should be in place to assure quality care.

Outcome

The outcome of home care represents the most direct measure of quality. Important outcomes for children and their families include how family members are functioning under the constraints and opportunities of home care. Relevant measures include the impact of the child's health condition on the family (in terms of family economics, interpersonal activities, or mental health), how the primary parental caregivers and siblings are coping, and how the child is functioning. Standardized ways to assess such outcomes can help family members take stock of progress, identify areas in which help is needed, and learn how the child's abilities have changed over time.

Recent work has both improved the ability to measure outcomes and increased the recognition that outcomes are broader than simply the health and medical status of the child. The Medical Outcomes Study (Tarlov et al., 1989), focusing mainly on adults, defined four outcome categories: (1) medical or physical outcomes, (2) satisfaction with care, (3) functional outcomes, and (4) psychological and social outcomes. For children especially, outcomes that reflect *family* or *household* status and functioning must be added to this list. New ways of measuring family impact and childhood physical functioning across disease categories have become available (Stein & Jessop, 1990; Stein & Riessman, 1980).

Older measures of psychological status of children at times labeled youngsters with chronic illnesses as psychologically unhealthy because particular responses associated with illness symptoms were considered psychological problems (Perrin, Stein, & Drotar, 1991). Newer methods of measuring psychological function and resilience, independent of factors confounded by disease states (Walker, Stein, Perrin, & Jessop, 1990), represent an important step toward measuring important outcomes for children with chronic health conditions. As the most direct measure of the effectiveness and quality of programs, outcomes should be the main focus of evaluation.

In spite of this progress, many disincentives to assessing outcomes persist. Obstacles include (1) the lengthy time frame that the commitment to home care represents; (2) the multitude of providers, both professionals and lay caregivers such as family members or friends; (3) the difficulty of assigning responsibility for outcomes in the face of lengthy time frames and multiple providers; (4) the question of control (in contrast to the hospital where providers can more effectively control treatment); and (5) the unwillingness to be held accountable when control is not absolute and providers are many (Kane, 1991). These obstacles notwithstanding, ignoring the outcomes of home care serves these children and their families poorly.

Developing the criteria to assess the outcome of care, finding staff to carry out the assessment, providing feedback, and making and implementing recommendations to improve outcomes are admittedly difficult tasks. Insofar as home care represents a major commitment of families, parents have the strongest incentives to assure that outcomes of home care are assessed. With the assistance of case managers or other providers, parents may be best able to assess the outcome of home care and to effect change based on the findings.

Parents can be instrumental in developing a written plan that defines explicit goals and means of measuring periodic outcomes. This plan is a useful tool to improve provider performance. The plan defines the needs of a child and family, sets goals of services, and outlines the specific methods proposed to achieve those goals. A plan that is shared among providers will likely improve coordination. For such a plan to be effective, it must be developed by the family, and child where appropriate, in collaboration with health professionals and other providers.

Model plans from the education system, the Individual Family Service Plan (IFSP) and the Individual Education Plan (IEP) of Public Laws 99–457 and 94–142, respectively, can be applied to improve the quality of care of children with complex medical conditions and their families. These written plans define a child's or family's services, milestones that are expected to be met, and services that will be provided and by whom. The IFSP and IEP models require family concurrence and provide for parental input in their definition; parents who disagree with the plans have grievance rights that are set out in law. Such a formalized approach to planning the care at home for a child and family offers one approach to improving quality of care.

The development of QUIGS (quality indicator groups) for the elderly may have application for children (Kramer, 1990). These measures combine assessment of the processes of care with outcomes such as functional status, health status, knowledge, family strain, unmet needs, satisfaction, and utilization to assess the quality of care for elderly home-care patients in selected diagnostic groups, such as pulmonary conditions, neurologic conditions, and IV infusion therapy. As these measures develop, their modification may make them suitable for children and families and provide a useful tool to assess outcomes of home care.

SUMMARY

Assessment of quality in health care is always complicated, and especially so in the provision of home care for severely ill children. Yet the many concerns expressed by families, providers, and agency personnel indicate the clear need to define and improve quality in both home- and community-based services for these children. It is important to assess and improve quality in an explicit fashion, and families must have the central role in defining and assessing quality. Much more work is needed in the development of methods to monitor and improve quality, but much existing work can be applied to the area of home care for children.

5

Costs of Care

The costs of caring for children in the home and community are high. Utilization of services far exceeds that of most other children, and the costs of services are often much greater than the costs of the usual services that children without apparent illness receive. Both the published data and the observations of the families we met concur that the amount of health services used by children at home with complex medical conditions is many times that of their able-bodied peers.

Parents' descriptions of their children's use of health services document extensive interactions with health care providers. The mother of two girls with von Willebrand's disease described almost daily trips to the hospital because one daughter or the other had a bleeding episode. The parents of a ventilator-dependent year-old girl described a care routine that included private duty nurses 19 hours each day, medications every two hours, frequent suctioning, and weekly physical therapy; visits to the pediatrician and hospital were infrequent because of the youngster's stable condition. The mother of a teenage boy with chronic renal failure described her son's ongoing health care encounters—dialysis, nephrologist, surgeon, psychiatrist, general pediatrician, home-care nurse. These family stories are unique to the individual circumstances, but the stories repeat the general theme of frequent encounters with health services. The health care system is an integral part of these families' lives, and at times the frequency of contact exceeds those of more "ordinary" family activities such as grocery shopping or classroom visits.

Home-care costs for the elderly have been studied more thoroughly than the comparable costs for children. To a degree, lessons from the elderly can be extrapolated to home care for children; yet, as noted in Chapter 1, the goals, activities, and financial base for children differ substantially from those for the aged. The discussion that follows is limited by the meager financial data about home care for children and in fact provides a case for the importance of collecting much better data in the future.

Replacing hospital care with home care offers many advantages to families, hospitals, and insurers. Children and families are reunited in the caring environment of the home. Hospitals are able to reduce financial losses that they may incur by providing lengthy, costly care to children with complex health disorders whose care is inadequately financed. Insurers save money because they usually pay less for home care than for hospital care. Nonetheless, home care may not save money for society. High-quality home care is very expensive, and much of the expense is borne by families who give up jobs or reduce work hours to care for their children and then provide that care without compensation. Hospital costs may decrease, but reductions are achieved by shifting much of the burden of expense from the hospital to the family.

USE AND COSTS OF HEALTH SERVICES BY CHILDREN WITH LONG-TERM HEALTH CONDITIONS: GENERAL POPULATION STUDIES

Use of Health Services

Studies at community and national levels confirm the greater use of health services by children with chronic conditions. With a sample drawn from a university medical center's clinics of children with cystic fibrosis, cerebral palsy, myelodysplasia, or multiple handicaps, Smyth-Staruch and colleagues (1984) found health service utilization many times that of a stratified, randomly sampled comparison group (Table 5–1).

Chronically ill children make much greater use of all services except dental care; they have 2.7 times as many doctor's visits, 14.5 times as many hospital days, and 240 times as many physical therapy treatments.

An analysis of the 1980 National Medical Care Utilization and Expenditure Survey (NMCUES) compared health service utilization of children under 21 with limitations in activity (play, school, or work depending on age) to those without limitations (Newacheck & McManus, 1988). Children with activity limitations used health services more than twice as frequently as did their peers without limitations (Table 5–2). These findings are consistent with those of the Smyth-Staruch study, although the differences are less dramatic.

Direct Costs of Long-Term Childhood Illness

The following sections examine the costs of long-term childhood illness, first for the general population of children with complex conditions and then for specific diseases. We review both the direct cost of health services and the additional costs to families related to decreased opportunity to seek gainful

Table 5-1. Comparison of Use of Health Services by Children with Chronic Conditions and Comparison Group

Service (Average use per child per year)	Children with chronic conditions	Comparison group
Hospital days	5.8	0.4
Doctor's visits	8.9	3.3
Dental visits	1.8	2.5
Occupational therapy treatments	12.0	0
Physical therapy treatments	24.0	0.1
Speech therapy visits	17.4	1.1
Mental health/social service visits	3.3	0.6
Psychiatrist or psychologist visits	0.27	0.03
Counselor visits	0.8	0.5

Source: Smyth-Staruch et al., 1984.

employment. Few studies have carefully collected and documented the costs that are incurred in caring for children with complex medical conditions, and the data here reflect a sparse literature. Despite these limitations, the reports consistently describe the high costs of care for children in home care—those who are technology-dependent as well as those who require extensive treatment and therapy by parents or other family members.

Increased use of health services leads to higher costs for both insurers and families and increases the amount of uncompensated care for children without insurance or other resources. Costs of care for children with chronic conditions are substantially greater than are costs incurred by able-bodied children. Families with children with one of ten long-term health conditions estimated the medical and nonmedical expenses incurred by their children during 1987

Table 5-2. Comparison of the Use of Health Services by Children with Limitation in Activity and Those with No Limitation

Health services	Limitation in activity	No limitation
Hospital admissions (per 1000)	269.0	123.5
Hospital days (per 1000)	1739.1	441.9
Average number of doctor's visits (per child)	5.1	2.8
Average number of visits to nonphysician providers	5.5	0.9
Average number of prescribed medications	4.0	2.0
Average, other medical items	0.4	0.2

Source: Newacheck & McManus, 1988.

(General Accounting Office, 1989). Of the families that estimated average monthly expenses, 34 percent reported total expenses less than $250 a month ($3000 per year), whereas 66 percent reported monthly expenses above this level.

Newacheck and McManus (1988) documented in more detail the greater costs for children with activity limitations in 1980. Average total charges for health services were $760, and out-of-pocket expenses incurred by their families averaged $135. In contrast, average total charges for an able-bodied comparison group were $263, and out-of-pocket expenses were $76. Furthermore, charges for children with limitations in activity are highly skewed. The top 10 percent of children accounted for 65 percent of all charges; the top 25 percent incurred 87 percent of total charges. Similarly, the top 10 percent of children incurred 63 percent of all out-of-pocket payments; the top quartile incurred 85 percent. Within the top decile, out-of-pocket payments exceeded $300.

Other analyses of 1980 NMCUES data demonstrated that $345 was spent per capita on the health care of all children under age 19 years (Butler, Winter, Singer, & Wenger, 1985b). Comparing this amount with the $760 average total charges in 1980 for health services for children with limitations in activity found by Newacheck and McManus (1988) confirms the greater health care expenses of children with health problems.

These health care costs are only a small portion of the total extra costs incurred by families with children with complex medical conditions. They include usual medical care costs such as hospital or physician services, medications, and specialized therapies, but this accounting leaves out additional hidden costs and nonmedical expenses. Transportation for doctors' visits and hospital stays, increased electric bills for powering necessary equipment, and home modifications to prepare the home and a room for the child are a few of these hidden costs.

Opportunity Costs

Opportunity costs (the income lost from the inability to make use of certain opportunities such as employment) are rarely documented but wreak havoc with family finances and undermine parental self-esteem. Opportunity cost may be defined as "the value of the good or service forgone" (Samuelson & Nordhaus, 1989, p.33). Opportunity costs include employment lost so that a parent can stay home to provide care, raises that are refused to enable a family to continue eligibility for benefits tied to family income, and job transfers or promotions that are turned down to prevent the family from losing insurance coverage.

Opportunity costs are often difficult to quantify. One mother described restricting her employment to half-time and her income to less than $10,000 so that her son with hemophilia would be eligible for Medicaid (Hemophilia Center). Most of these opportunity costs have never been estimated, although a few, such as the effects of chronically ill children on the labor force participation of mothers, have been studied.

Using the 1972 National Health Interview Survey, Salkever (1982) studied how the presence of a disabled child in the family affected the mother's participation in the work force. He found that in white, two-parent families, mothers with a disabled child worked outside the home about 10 percent less than did mothers without disabled children. A similar study compared work force participation of mothers of children with specific chronic illnesses (cystic fibrosis, cerebral palsy, myelodysplasia, and multiple physical handicaps) with that of mothers of children with no disabilities (Breslau, Salkever, & Staruch, 1982). Mothers of chronically ill children, especially those at low income levels, participated less in the work force.

A related study by Breslau (1983) compared time spent on household work (for example, cooking and cleaning) and child care. As compared with controls, married mothers of chronically ill children spent nearly four additional hours each week on household chores. No significant differences were found in time spent in child care. However, home therapy provided by parents required an average of 6.9 hours weekly for those children for whom therapy was recommended. Families of chronically ill children also spent more time on visits to doctors than did families of able-bodied children. The increased number of visits annually (9 versus 3) combined with the greater amount of time per visit (127 minutes versus 51 minutes) and the longer travel time to the site (38.4 minutes versus 17.6 minutes, respectively) resulted in families of chronically ill children devoting 30.6 hours each year for visits to doctors as compared with 4.75 hours yearly for families with able-bodied children.

Those parents of chronically ill children who do participate in the labor force must also address the child's home nursing care needs during an acute illness or exacerbation of the chronic condition. General population estimates are that women working full-time outside the home, on average, miss an additional seven workdays each year because a child's illness (Carpenter, 1980). Increased school absence for chronic illness is well documented; and these school absences likely result in more parental absence from work. In Scandinavian countries, parents of children with chronic conditions receive extra paid leave from work because society recognizes the increased time demands of children with special health needs (Personal communication, Dr. Bengt Zachau-Christiansen, 1982).

COSTS OF SPECIFIC HEALTH CONDITIONS

National data clarify average costs of caring for children with disabilities but shed little light on the personal experiences of families whose children have chronic illnesses. National data often obscure the great variations in financial burden that families shoulder when raising a child with a complex medical condition. Some families, and especially those who provide extensive home care, are at the high end of the spectrum and carry extraordinary expenses. Reports of costs for different chronic illnesses reflect the idiosyncracies of each illness. Comparison across illnesses is made more difficult because studies rarely include the same expenses in their analyses. Nevertheless, information and data gathered from published reports and from advocacy groups that focus on specific health conditions provide an overview of the expenses faced by families.

The studies from which the costs by condition were derived were published over a period of nearly 20 years. To improve comparability, we adjusted the dollar amounts in the examples that follow in this chapter, unless otherwise noted, to 1988 dollars. Adjustments were made from the year of publication of the study using the consumer price indexes, 1960–1988 (U.S. Department of Labor, 1990), either for the "medical care index" or "all items" as appropriate. Arithmetic adjustments of this type cannot account for therapeutic advances that may have substantially altered the cost of care.

The following reports document medical costs, nonmedical costs, and opportunity costs for specific medical conditions. Medical care costs include the costs of physician and surgeon services, hospital care, home nursing care, physical, occupational and speech and language therapies, medications, and medical supplies and equipment. Nonmedical costs include transportation, lodging, food, babysitting, parking, clothes, and diapers.

Ventilator-Dependent Children

Reports of the costs of caring for ventilator-dependent children (and others dependent on similar high-tech care) typically limit their focus to the child's medical expenses and ignore other costs that families incur. Staggering expenses of home care, $1850 to $138,785 annually in 1980 in Massachusetts, are still considerably less than the cost of care in the hospital, which ranged from $257,600 to $741,200 during the same year (1980 dollars adjusted to 1988) (Burr et al., 1983). More recent reports indicate a similar magnitude of reduction in costs. Average yearly costs of hospital care in Maryland in 1986 (dollars adjusted to 1988 levels) of nearly $341,000 compare with home-care costs of $125,000. Similar comparisons in Louisiana indicate hospital care costs of $354,000 and home-care costs of $41,000. Hospital costs in Illinois varied by payer source; annual Medicaid costs averaged $232,000, while costs for private insurers averaged $362,000. The costs at home were similar for both payers, averaging $86,000 for Medicaid and $94,000 for private payers (U.S. Congress, 1987). Similar cost savings have been shown for adults who have returned home with ventilator support (Banaszak et al., 1981; Sivak et al., 1983).

Reported cost savings attributable to home care, especially for ventilator-dependent and other technology-dependent youngsters, have been fabricated to some extent as a result of funding requirements. Most insurers (public and private) require that home care for technology-dependent children be less costly than institutional care. As a result, family service plans are developed with this financial limitation in mind, and figures may be manipulated to demonstrate that home care is much less expensive than hospital care. Much of the reported savings results from care and room and board provided by families for which they receive no compensation—all costs that are paid when a child is in a hospital (Frates et al., 1985). The savings to insurers might be substantial. For instance, an insurer might pay $550 a day for hospital care that includes nursing services and room and board as compared with nothing for the same services provided by the family. Care provided in the home by a nurse or aide may offset the daily savings, but even with 16 hours of care at $20 an hour, the insurer saves $230 each day, all at the expense of the family.

Another portion of the savings comes from increased cost-sharing payments that families pay when the child returns home. Insurance policies that pay 100 percent of a hospital bill often pay only 80 percent for care provided in the home (Burr et al., 1983). Eighty-three percent of families caring for ventilator-dependent children at home incurred nonreimbursed expenses of $1000 or more in a year (Quint et al., 1990). Another mother described the financial disincentive for home care for her ventilator-dependent child: "The thing was, she was covered 100 percent in the hospital. Up until we left and came home. It's as though they don't want these children to come home" (Thorp, 1987, p. 139)

Cancer

The costs of cancer, both in the short term for the duration of intensive treatment and in the long term for the survivor, can be staggering. Strayer, Kisker, and Fethke (1980) compared community-based treatment with standard treatment at an academic medical center. This study documented both direct medical care costs and some hidden costs as well as the savings that can result from receiving care closer to home. The two treatment groups experienced similar medical care costs (visits to doctors, laboratory fees, drugs and their administration): $3627 for children receiving care at the academic medical center as compared with $3496 for children cared for by community pediatricians. But families whose children received community-based care faced substantially lower nonmedical costs (transportation, parking, meals away from home), costs that most families pay out-of-pocket at the time they are incurred: $722 for community-based care as compared with $2083 for academic medical center care.

The study also examined opportunity costs. Both groups of families faced considerable lost wages, but these were more moderate for families receiving community-based care: $1156 rather than $2840. The total amounts incurred by parents, including nonmedical and opportunity costs, were $1878 for community-based care and $4923 for care at the academic medical center. Most families pay additional amounts for deductibles and co-payments before insurance covers their child's medical expenses. These totals yield an enormous expense that few families can easily absorb.

Lansky and others (1979) reported nonmedical expenses and opportunity costs for a similar group of families with children with cancer. Average weekly nonmedical expenses, including meals, lodging, transportation, babysitters, clothes, and miscellaneous items, totalled $91.30. Average opportunity costs each week came to $65.13. Applying these expenses over the 16-month time frame that the Strayer study found to be the typical length of treatment results in average nonmedical and opportunity costs to the family of $6330 and $4515, respectively, and total expenses of $10,845. These amounts, which again exclude that portion of direct medical expenses that the family may be required to pay, are well beyond the means of most families and create a catastrophic burden.

Average annual medical expenses, non-medical expenses, and opportunity costs for the care of children with cancer treated at Children's Hospital of Philadelphia in 1981 were $25,839 for inpatient care, $6363 for outpatient services, and $12,737 for out-of-pocket expenses (dollars adjusted from 1981) (Bloom et al., 1985). Out-of-pocket expenses were further separated into one-time costs (such as special equipment, 9.5 percent of total), continuing costs (such as travel expenses, 31.5 percent), medical costs (10.8 percent), and lost wages (48.1 percent). With an average income of $33,798 in this group of families, the out-of-pocket expense of $12,737 was surely catastrophic. This magnitude of expense, difficult enough to absorb in a single year, is an ongoing cost that families with children with cancer incur for the duration of treatment and follow-up. Although some families, through savings and the help of extended family, may be able to cover such a huge expense for a single year, few families can remain financially secure and continue to incur this level of out-of-pocket cost on an ongoing basis.

A hidden cost of cancer treatment is revealed when the childhood survivor attempts to get health or life insurance as an adult. Some 24 percent of survivors of childhood cancer reported difficulty getting health insurance as compared with a matched sample of siblings, none of whom reported problems (Holmes et al., 1986). Most survivors succeeded in finding health insurance; nevertheless, survivors were twice as likely to lack insurance as their matched adult siblings. Similarly, 44 percent of cancer survivors reported problems when they sought life insurance. Again, cancer survivors were more than twice as likely to lack life insurance. The stigma of childhood cancer lingers far beyond treatment and follows a survivor well into adulthood.

Cystic Fibrosis

McCollum (1971) examined medical care costs for cystic fibrosis in a 1968–1969 survey of 54 families with 62 affected children. Average annual costs were $4703, but the median cost was $2377. The skewed distribution of expenses resulted from the tremendous cost for children who were hospitalized. The 51 children who required only outpatient treatment had average costs of $2315; the 11 children who were hospitalized averaged $15,784. Added to these medical costs were an average $2526 for medical care outside the medical center, expenses related to clinic visits, pulmonary therapy, and extra food. Costs for transportation, insurance premiums, home health visits, or lost pay were not included. With an average gross family income of $28,334, these expenses easily reached catastrophic levels.

A 1980 Cystic Fibrosis Foundation survey of adults with cystic fibrosis further describes the costs of care for this condition (Cystic Fibrosis Foundation, 1980). Over half of the adults responding to the survey reported no inpatient stays in the previous year, but those who were hospitalized had an average of 21 inpatient days during 2.2 admissions. Median annual medical costs were $3954 for respondents who had not been hospitalized in the past year, and $17,555 for those who had. Seventy-eight percent of those responding to the survey had at least 70 percent of medical expenses paid by insurance; but 22 percent remained personally responsible for costly medical bills.

Cystic fibrosis in an adult imposes additional costs related to employment. The survey respondents reported an unemployment rate of 16.7 percent, and half of those who were unemployed listed their health condition as the reason. Of those who were employed, one-third worked part-time rather than full-time because of their health. The employed respondents reported a median of 10.5

days lost from work in the previous year. A quarter of the respondents felt that they had experienced job discrimination because of their health condition.

Recent advances in home administration of antibiotics offer special advantages to people with cystic fibrosis who experience pulmonary flare-ups that require IV antibiotic administration. A randomized controlled trial of home administration of IV therapy for children and young adults with cystic fibrosis in the mid-1980s demonstrated that home treatment is safe and effective (Donati, Guenette, & Auerbach, 1987). Costs for home treatment, $10,661, were substantially lower than the $19,191 cost for hospital care. The additional advantages of home care included avoiding a hospital stay with the risk of hospital-acquired infections and the opportunity to maintain normal community activities such as work and school.

Chronic Kidney Disease

Full costs of caring for children with end-stage renal disease have not been reported. However, Hoffstein and colleagues (1976) reported dialysis treatment costs for 1973. Reported annual costs (adjusted from 1973) ranged from $24,037 for self-care at home to $59,012 for out-of-hospital, center-based care. These costs ignore substantial additional direct medical expenses (for example, physicians' services). A family's report of expenses between 1973 and 1977 for care of an adult with chronic renal failure noted total costs for dialysis and transplantation of $108,548, $16,148 of which was paid out-of-pocket for nonmedical needs (for example, premiums, transportation, moving) (Campbell & Campbell, 1978). This report of an adult's confrontation with renal failure reflects similar problems for families with children with chronic illness.

The average annual cost for a child under age 15 in the Medicare End Stage Renal Disease Program is $28,400 (unadjusted dollars). This amount includes all medical expenses that would be covered by Medicare (for example, dialysis sessions, fees to physicians, medications, and hospitalizations) (Personal communication, Paul Eggers, 1991). However, costs such as foods for special diets will not be covered by Medicare and must be absorbed by the family.

Hemophilia

Hemophilia is a condition for which a technological breakthrough, the production of factor concentrates that can be administered at home, has had a major, positive effect on home care and outcomes of care for patients and families. Notable decreases in days lost from school or work (14.5 to 4.3), in rates of hospital admissions annually (1.9 to 0.26), and in unemployment of adults (36 percent to 12.8 percent) have been reported (Smith & Levine, 1984). Family out-of-pocket expenses decreased from $1106 to $445 while overall costs of care dropped from $26,416 to $9,918 (1981 figures adjusted to 1988).

The risk of transfusion-induced HIV infection now jeopardizes the gains achieved from home administration of clotting factor. To reduce the risk, manufacturers of blood products are increasing production of high-purity clotting factor concentrates that eliminate HIV and hepatitis viruses. However, such clotting factor is much more costly to produce. As more expensive, high-purity factor replaces less costly, intermediate-purity factor, people with hemophilia who already have HIV infection will be unnecessarily forced to pay a higher price for treatment. Aledort and colleagues (1988) recommend that manufacturers be given immunity to encourage them to continue to make the lower-cost intermediate-purity factor.

The National Hemophilia Foundation has documented the huge cost increase for treating boys with hemophilia (National Hemophilia Foundation Bulletins, 1989–1991). Manufacturers attribute the price increases to new production methods that are more costly and less efficient than previously employed techniques that produced lower purity blood products. Extraordinary increases were documented from 1987 to 1988 for new clotting factor that replaced previously available factor (increases ranging from 617 percent to 829 percent); but substantial increases were also experienced in the absence of costly production changes (up to a 192 percent increase per unit). Because of more costly production techniques and reduced supplies, annual costs for treating some boys with hemophilia have risen to as much as $100,000.

Increased costs for treating hemophilia have been reluctantly borne by insurers who are not convinced of the need for treatment with high purity factor. The National Hemophilia Foundation advocated with the Health Care Financing Administration for improved inpatient reimbursement for care of Medicare recipients with hemophilia, and in April 1990 new reimbursement regulations were announced. This breakthrough with Medicare will likely influence the reimbursement decisions of other insurers, increasing the likelihood that they too will pay for the increased cost of treatment.

Rheumatologic Diseases

McCormick and others (1986) surveyed 138 families of children with rheumatologic diseases about the impact of these conditions on family life. Some 27.5 percent of families reported one or more hospital admissions in the previous year, and 58.7 percent had one or more physician visits in the past month. Two-thirds of the hospitalized children's parents incurred out-of-pocket expenses averaging $591; over half of these families reported difficulty paying this bill. Other medical expenses reported by the families included supplies, parking fees, and physical therapy.

Meningomyelocele

Costs of direct treatment for meningomyelocele, a condition also known as spina bifida that results from improper closure of the spinal column during fetal life, were reported in 1974 and updated in 1979 (McLaughlin & Shurtleff, 1979; Shurtleff et al., 1974). Reported expenses did not include the cost of therapies or services paid directly by families. Even with these exclusions, costs of treatment for the first six years of life were high. Costs varied with the level of the lesion and ranged from $24,333 for a sacral (low spinal) lesion, $42,320 for an L3–5 (mid-back) lesion, to $50,248 for a lesion at L2 and above (upper back). These costs mainly reflect medical and surgical treatments and also include the cost of institutional or foster care required by some children. These costs significantly understate the ongoing expenses borne by families for nonmedical needs and for treatment of youngsters beyond age six.

The estimated (lifetime) total costs (1985 dollars) for a child with meningomyelocele are $250,000 and include medical care, long-term care, disability, education, and indirect costs such as reduced productivity and loss of parental wages (Centers for Disease Control, 1989). The Spina Bifida Association contends that the Center for Disease Control (CDC) estimates vastly understate the expenses experienced by parents in its membership. The association estimates that most families incur $250,000 of expenses by the time the child with spina bifida reaches his or her eighth birthday and that expenses through age 13 are commonly $500,000.

Many incidental medical expenses, not covered by insurance, and nonmedical expenses were reported by the father of a young man, a high school senior, with spina bifida. Purchase of crutches ($60–$100), treatment of skin breakdown ($20 a day), catheters, diapers, wheelchairs for athletics, and hand controls for the family car are examples of expenses that insurance will not pay. Extra costs for special pants with elastic waists for people in wheelchairs, special trips to see colleges to determine handicapped accessibility before applying, and increased carpooling responsibilities because theirs was the only car that would accommodate a wheelchair are examples of some of the hidden, nonmedical expenses absorbed by this family. These extra out-of-pocket expenses, while specific to one family's experience with a son with spina bifida, can be applied to others whose children have impairments of mobility (Personal communication, Spina Bifida Association parent, March 1991).

SUMMARY

Health care for children with complex medical conditions is two to three times more costly than care for able-bodied children. For children with long-term health conditions, expenses for medical care, nonmedical services, and opportunity costs are borne by society as well as by families. Clearly, the expenses incurred by parents of a boy with hemophilia differ greatly from those experienced by a family whose daughter has juvenile rheumatoid arthritis or by the parents of a ventilator-dependent child. Nevertheless, all conditions impose considerable expenses, including at least medical care costs that are paid by insurance, by the family (for deductibles, co-insurance requirements, direct payments for uninsured services, and so forth), and by providers through uncompensated care. Services that are not covered create extra costs to the family. These additional expenses encompass nonmedical items (for example, babysitters for siblings; parking; lodging near the hospital; telephone calls), and opportunity costs such as lost wages or offers of paid employment that have to be refused.

Caring for a chronically ill child at home imposes many costs not encountered by most other families. Families face increased telephone bills; higher utility bills for heating, air conditioning, or operating supportive equipment; expenditures for extra clothing or special furnishings; a second car; home modifications; babysitters; and special diets. These costs, rarely paid by insurance, represent a special burden for families because they must be paid out-of-pocket (usually at the time they are incurred), because they strain already thin budgets, and because they are regular expenses that families can expect to incur on an ongoing basis.

Opportunity costs borne by families of children with complex chronic conditions combined with the out-of-pocket costs that they incur in the care of their children impose a substantial added financial burden on young families. At a time when the peers of the parents are becoming more secure financially and can begin to save for a home, education, or other family needs, parents of most children with complex conditions still struggle to make ends meet.

With increased health care costs, extraordinary out-of-pocket expenditures, and greater opportunity costs, families with children with complex medical conditions are likely to incur catastrophic expenses. Options for helping families to meet these expenses are reviewed in the next chapter.

6

Paying for Care

Sources of payment for services for children with complex medical conditions include private health insurance, public financing programs such as Medicaid and the Title V Program for Children with Special Health Care Needs, and school programs through the Education of the Handicapped Act of 1975 and its revisions. These several programs, although providing an important base of financing, leave many families without any source of payment at all and many more with only partial coverage. The main options currently considered for filling gaps in coverage include catastrophic insurance, high risk pools, and universal health insurance programs.

The United States finances health care for children through a variety of unrelated programs. Virtually all of the elderly in America have identical basic coverage for health expenses through the single federal program Medicare. In contrast, children's health care is financed from multiple sources, including federal-state partnerships (mainly Medicaid and the Title V Program for Children with Special Health Care Needs), parents' employers (group health coverage), insurance directly purchased by the family, out-of-pocket payment, or from charity care resulting from nonpayment. Only the few children who are enrolled in Medicare through the End-Stage Renal Disease Program and in the Civilian Health and Medical Program of the United States (CHAMPUS) receive consistent, federally provided coverage. With these multiple financing programs, many children slip through the holes in the financing system; in 1987, 19.4 percent of children under 18 were without health insurance (McManus & Greaney, 1988). This chapter describes the child health financing programs most relevant to the home care of children with severe illnesses: Medicaid, private insurance, prepaid group practice, the Title V Program for Children with Special Health Care Needs, and the Education of the Handicapped Act of 1975.

MEDICAID

Medicaid, dating to 1965, has its roots in state welfare systems; as such, although it springs from federal legislation, it is an amalgam of individual state programs. In 1988, an estimated 11.1 million youngsters under age 21 were eligible for Medicaid (U.S. Department of Health and Human Services, 1989). Federal guidelines require Medicaid programs to serve the poor, the disabled, and the aged; but states have great latitude within broad federal guidelines in establishing eligibility requirements and benefits. State Medicaid eligibility for children is largely tied to enrollment in Aid to Families with Dependent Children (AFDC or welfare) and hence to family finances; families risk losing coverage as incomes rise. Over the course of a year, fully one-third of families on Medicaid lose their coverage for one reason or another. Although states must provide a set of basic benefits, they may offer optional benefits at their discretion; and states may apply limitations to all benefits, both mandatory and optional. Depending on the states' choices regarding eligibility and benefits, the Medicaid program can be a rich resource with great depth and breadth of services or more impoverished, meeting only minimal needs for the poorest of the poor. The great interstate variation in eligibility criteria and benefits creates major inequities in the Medicaid program.

Eligibility

Two main factors determine eligibility for Medicaid: disability and financial status. A disabled child meeting income and disability criteria for Supplemental Security Income (SSI), the federal program of cash assistance for aged, blind, or disabled people, is eligible for Medicaid in most states. The SSI program currently serves relatively few children; in 1990, approximately 290,000 youngsters received SSI benefits, most of whom were eligible for Medicaid (Fox & Greaney, 1988). Eligibility for children has been limited until recently by difficulty in determining the functional abilities of very young children with disabilities, in accounting for additive effects of multiple handicaps, and in dealing with the many rare conditions that disable youngsters. As a result of a U.S. Supreme Court ruling in early 1990 (*Sullivan v. Zebley*), the Social Security Administration developed new regulations to ease the eligibility determination process for children. Approximately two-thirds of childhood recipients of SSI benefits prior to the Supreme Court decision were children with mental retardation and certain diseases of the central nervous system, with relatively few having other forms of chronic health impairments. The new regulations will likely improve access of many children with other types of physical disabilities to SSI benefits. Current estimates are that the program may grow by 50 to 100 percent in numbers of childhood beneficiaries, depending on the methods of implementing the new regulations (Perrin & Stein, 1991). The size of the SSI financial benefit depends on family income and on the state of residence, insofar as many states supplement the federal payment. With the Medicaid eligibility that accompanies SSI enrollment in most states, SSI provides a valuable financial benefit for families.

The second main avenue for Medicaid eligibility, through enrollment in the Aid to Families with Dependent Children (AFDC) program, requires meeting family structure guidelines and state-specific income need standards. States have vastly different income standards to determine AFDC (and therefore Medicaid) eligibility. Maximum allowable monthly income in 1985–1986 ranged from $208 for a family of four in New Mexico to $943 for a similar family in Vermont (U.S. Department of Health and Human Services, 1987).

The optional medically needy program provides another route for Medicaid eligibility. This program provides Medicaid coverage for people who meet the "categorical" requirements for Medicaid (i.e., have family structure or disability like other AFDC recipients) and have income not exceeding 133 percent of the maximum AFDC payment set by the states. In addition, similar families whose incomes exceed this ceiling but whose medical expenses will offset the excess income are also eligible for Medicaid through the "spend down" provision. Although this program, available in 35 states as of 1986, offers great potential to meet the needs of children with complex medical conditions, its arcane administration provides substantial barriers to enrollment.

A second optional Medicaid program, targeted to children and pregnant women, was first enacted as part of the Omnibus Budget Reconciliation Act (OBRA) of 1986. This program provides Medicaid coverage to pregnant women and to children under age 5, regardless of family structure, whose income is below the *federal* poverty standard. This change represents a major break in the link between Medicaid and AFDC. Families no longer need to be eligible for welfare benefits to receive Medicaid (Pear, 1988). In 1987, OBRA further permitted Medicaid enrollment of pregnant women who had incomes up to 185 percent of the poverty level and who had infants under 1 year of age; also eligible are children up to age 8 whose family income is below the federal poverty level. Moreover, OBRA in 1987 *required* Medicaid coverage of children up to age 7, regardless of family structure, whose family income was less than the state's AFDC need standard (Newacheck, 1988; Rosenbaum, 1988). Further Medicaid amendments that took effect in 1990 *mandated* that states provide Medicaid to children up to age 6 and all pregnant women with incomes below 133 percent of the federal poverty level. This was an effort to improve access to health care and to develop national standards for eligibility.

These expansions provide coverage for needy women and children and offer another important route for medically complex youngsters to receive coverage for medical expenses.

Benefits

All states must offer basic health care benefits (subject to certain limitations) and have the option of providing others. Nevertheless, states have much leeway in what their Medicaid benefit package includes. Required basic benefits especially relevant to children with chronic health conditions include inpatient hospital services, outpatient hospital services, rural health clinics (if allowed under state law), other laboratory and X-ray services, Early Periodic Screening, Diagnosis, and Treatment (EPSDT) program services, family planning, physicians' services, home health services, and nurse-midwife services (if midwife practice is permitted under state law). Optional services include prescription drugs; transportation; personal-care services; private duty nursing; optometry; eyeglasses; dental services; physical and occupational therapies; and speech, hearing, and language services. The EPSDT program, especially through the treatment component and some administrative provisions, expands coverage and services beyond the limits of the regular Medicaid program to children whose conditions were identified as part of an EPSDT visit. The OBRA 1989 Medicaid expansions now require states to provide the full range of federally approved Medicaid services (even if these services are not included in the state's Medicaid plan) to treat children whose conditions were identified through an EPSDT visit. An additional OBRA 1989 provision authorizes health care providers to give "partial" EPSDT screening exams (Fox, 1990); this provision may undermine the comprehensiveness of services for some children but offers the advantage to many others, especially youngsters with complex medical conditions, to enhance care coordination by paying primary-care providers for both regular exams and EPSDT screens. Many elements of these benefit packages can greatly enhance health care opportunities for severely ill children under Medicaid.

States' choices of benefits under Medicaid yield vastly different programs. A comparison of coverage in two states in 1986 demonstrates the effect of these choices. A Medicaid-eligible child with chronic illness residing in Massachusetts has access to a rich plan of benefits. The state Medicaid program provides inpatient hospital days, outpatient hospital visits, home health visits, home health aides, home-care services (physical and occupational therapies, speech and hearing), and prescription drugs with no limitations on use or number of visits. However, limits are applied to private duty nursing, transportation, physical and occupational therapy, and speech therapy. The same child living in Tennessee has sharply curtailed coverage. Restricted utilization applies to all services that are unlimited in Massachusetts: There are 14 inpatient days per year, 30 outpatient visits per year, 24 doctor's office visits per year, and limitations on all home-care services and prescriptions. Other services, limited in Massachusetts, are not provided at all (U.S. Department of Health and Human Services, 1987). The differences in generosity of Medicaid benefits in these two states yield different results. The child with chronic illness in Massachusetts will likely have most medical needs met and face only a few gaps in service. In contrast, peers in Tennessee will go without many needed services, while unavoidable but uncovered services (for example, hospitalization in excess of 14 days per year) will be provided as unpaid, charity care from local institutions.

Waivers and Amendments

While the value of Medicaid is undeniable, the remaining problems are equally glaring. Vastly different need standards, limited benefits, on-and-off coverage with small fluctuations in family income, intrusive family structure requirements, and endless bureaucratic red tape are just a few of the problems that plague this important program. State Medicaid programs, when implemented with creativity and compassion, offer real opportunities for serving children with chronic health conditions. Two options in particular, Medicaid waiver programs and state amendments to Medicaid plans through the Tax Equity and Fiscal Responsibility Act of 1982 (TEFRA), offer great promise for helping families care for complex chronically ill children at home.

The Medicaid waiver programs began in 1982 as the result of advocacy by Julianne Beckett, the mother of Katie Beckett. Mrs. Beckett bristled at the inflexibility of the Medicaid program that covered Katie after she had exhausted her private insurance benefits but still remained hospitalized. Medicaid would pay Katie's medical expenses if she stayed in the hospital but would not continue to cover her if she returned home and had substantially lower, although still considerable, expenses. Without Medicaid coverage, the middle-income Becketts could not afford to bring their medically complex daughter home from the hospital.

Rather than simply complain about the situation, Mrs. Beckett lobbied public officials until she finally reached her representative in Congress. He brought this situation to the attention of then-Vice President George Bush, and President Ronald Reagan then directed that something be done to correct the problem. Thus was born the Katie Beckett waiver program that operated from 1982 until 1984.

Katie Beckett waivers permitted individual exceptions to Medicaid's income-deeming requirements so that severely ill, hospitalized children would be able to return home and still maintain Medicaid coverage if their families could document cost savings and appropriate quality with home care. Children who had been granted Katie Beckett waivers have remained in the Beckett program, but these individual waivers are no longer issued. Instead, Section 2176 of the 1981 Omnibus Budget Reconciliation Act authorized Home- and Community-Based Services Waivers to replace the individual waivers.

Medicaid waiver programs allow approved states to forgo certain Medicaid requirements (for example, income standards for eligibility, deeming rules, and freedom of choice of providers) or to provide additional benefits as long as home care is safe and costs to the Medicaid program will not increase. Section 2176 of the Home- and Community-Based Services Waivers includes two types of programs: the "regular" waivers that permit an unlimited number of enrollees and the "model" waivers that are limited to 200 individuals. The Section 2176 waivers allow states to offer expanded services to targeted recipients (aged, disabled, mentally retarded, mentally ill) so as to avoid more costly institutionalization. Additional services allowed through a waiver (beyond the state's usual Medicaid services) include case management, homemakers, home health aides, personal-care services, adult day care, habilitation, respite care, private-duty nursing, and home modification (Fox, 1984; Hall, 1990).

The Section 2176 waiver programs have the potential to improve financing and services for children with complex medical conditions. As of 1989, some 36 states were approved for a total of 66 waivers that serve children. Of these 66 waivers, 42 are regular waivers and 24 are model waivers (Hall, 1990). The value of the waiver to families of complex, chronically ill children is substantial. Children who, in the absence of the waiver, would have stayed in hospital to remain on Medicaid now live at home with their families and still keep their coverage. Moreover, the additional services available through the waivers help families to cope long term with the stress of a medically complex child at home.

Nevertheless, the waivers fall short of meeting the needs of many families. Model waivers are limited to 200 individuals regardless of the population of the state, so the needs of the 201st child and all subsequent children remain unmet in states where the waiver slots are filled. Under these circumstances, an additional waiver may be requested by the state. Waivers also fail to serve youngsters whose home care is more costly to Medicaid that their hospital care. This situation can arise when a child's hospital care is paid by private insurance that will not provide home-care benefits. In such a case, Medicaid is obligated to pay nothing for hospital care so that any home-care plan that would be paid by Medicaid would not meet the cost-effectiveness requirement.

States structure the waivers differently. Benefits vary substantially, both in their definition and in the amount of services that will be covered. Waivers require documentation that care at home will be less expensive than care in an institution. The comparison base for determining cost-effectiveness varies: Some states compare home costs with rates for acute-care hospitals whereas other states compare costs with rates at skilled nursing facilities (SNF). This seemingly minor difference allows waiver-approved children in acute-care-comparison states to justify vastly more comprehensive services than their peers in the SNF-comparison states because of the huge difference in the cost comparison threshold. In some states, parents transfer their children to more expensive hospitals so that it will be easier to show comparative cost savings with home care.

The differences between the model waivers of Iowa and Illinois illustrate these points. As of March 1986, the model waiver in Illinois provided funding for care management, respite care, home modifications, private-duty nursing, special medical supplies, and equipment and appliances; and the comparison basis for cost-effectiveness was the acute care hospital. With high-cost acute care serving as the economic ceiling, Illinois waiver families can "afford" great breadth and depth of services and can receive, for example, many hours of private-duty nursing to relieve the family's burden of care. In contrast, the Iowa waiver provides homemaker, home health aide, personal care, adult day care, respite care, and residential care and treatment services but uses skilled nursing facility rates as the basis for determining cost-effectiveness. The lower allowance for services in Iowa sharply curtails the benefits that families may receive under this program. An Iowa family with a child with major technological needs would be hard-pressed to bring the child home from the hospital with only Medicaid and waiver benefits to support home care.

Both waiver coverage and Medicaid coverage offer important benefits to avoid economic ruin and to assist families in caring for their children. Unfortunately, not all states offer waivers, and in the absence of community or other support, families in these areas endure great hardship to bring home medically complex children.

A 1986 study of model waivers that serve children documented the substantial cost savings realized by state Medicaid programs with the use of home care through the waivers (La Jolla Management Corporation, 1986). The average monthly cost saving (costs during the month prior to entry into the programs compared with three and six months after) was $3640. However, absolute costs and the savings realized with the use of the waiver varied widely with the type or severity of the child's condition. Technology-dependent children (for example, youngsters using ventilators or gastrostomy tubes) experienced the highest costs—$9100 monthly in hospital and $4500 monthly on home care with the waiver—while children with disorders of the central nervous system had significantly lower monthly costs both before and after home care—$3800 before and $1600 after. This study noted that waivers were infrequently used to expand funding options for children, and the authors recommended publicity to increase the visibility of waivers to the public and providers. They further recommended an expanded role for Title V agencies in the implementation of the waivers to assure quality of care, to advocate for the adoption of waivers by the states, to work with the Medicaid agencies to improve home care, and to provide case management with reimbursement from Medicaid.

Amendments to states' Medicaid plans authorized under Section 134 of the 1982 TEFRA act provide another option to serve the special needs of children with complex medical conditions. These TEFRA state plan options offer states the advantage of expanding eligibility for Medicaid benefits to certain populations within the state. This mechanism to expand Medicaid eligibility is easier administratively than applying for a waiver and has been selected in 17 states as of 1989 (Hall, 1990). This option for serving medically complex children is most beneficial in states that have a rich Medicaid program because the benefits are limited to those available through the regular program. Through this option, states may target Medicaid eligibility to certain needy groups without opening eligibility to a more general population. An amendment to the Medicaid plan in Massachusetts, the Kaileigh Mulligan Home Care for Disabled Children Program, is an example of such a special program, targeted to children with complex medical conditions.

The Kaileigh Mulligan program began with public pressure on the Massachusetts Department of Public Welfare to meet the medical needs of Kaileigh Mulligan, a child with multiple disabilities at home whose parents' income was above the Medicaid eligibility standard. The Kaileigh Mulligan program waives Medicaid financial needs standards if a child with a complex medical condition meets certain criteria: The child must be under age 19; must meet the Social Security Administration's criteria for disability for the SSI program; must require the level of care of an acute or chronic hospital or a pediatric nursing home (that is, the child is at risk of institutionalization but not necessarily residing in one); the child's personal assets and income must not exceed the maximum allowed for a child residing in an institution; home care must be less costly than the comparable institutional alternative; and home care must be safe and appropriate.

Under the Kaileigh Mulligan program, eligible children receive the rich benefits of the regular Medicaid program as well as case management services provided by the state's Title V program. As of December 1988, some 86 children were enrolled in the program. This program effectively relieves desperate home care situations for families.

One mother described her experiences before and after her son, who has a degenerative neurological condition, was accepted into the Kaileigh Mulligan program. When Mrs. Cameron spoke with us, James, 7 years old, required total care: He was able to vocalize but could not speak; his cognitive level was unmeasurable, and he was blind and had cerebral palsy, seizures, and spasticity. He required leg casts, a neck brace to support his enlarged head, a wheelchair, a suction machine, and a gastrostomy tube.

James's father was self-employed, and the family's costly health insurance policy with Blue Cross covered only minimal home-care benefits—one hour each week of nursing care and twice-weekly physical therapy. As James got older, his condition worsened, and his care requirements intensified. His parents advocated with the Department of Public Health for increased benefits, and his nursing hours were increased from 10 days for respite care every 6 months to 16 hours per week of home nursing care. In addition to these services, James attended an early intervention program since age 3, providing his mother a break from the burden of his care.

Following James's hospitalization for a second generalized seizure in January 1988 and short-term respirator support, Mrs. Cameron decided that the time had come to tackle the formidable Kaileigh Mulligan application. With James's acceptance into the Kaileigh Mulligan program and receipt of benefits, the Camerons received vastly increased nursing hours (60 hours weekly), formula for James's stomach tube, diapers, and a special seat to facilitate bathing. Mrs. Cameron admitted that these benefits made a world of difference to her and her husband, and she did not know how she would have survived without the additional home nursing care. Moreover, acceptance into the Kaileigh Mulligan program meant that, should James reach his $250,000 maximum lifetime benefits under his Blue Cross policy and lose his insurance coverage, he would not leave his parents responsible for paying for all his costly care.

PRIVATE HEALTH INSURANCE

The private health insurance system, including both commercial and Blue Cross/Blue Shield plans, pays for the majority of health care for children in the United States. In some cases, special benefits from private health insurance support home care for children with complex medical conditions, although there are many limitations of insurance in meeting family needs.

Private health insurance covered nearly 42 million youngsters (66.4 percent) under age 18 in the United States in 1986 (McManus & Greaney, 1988). Most health insurance coverage is provided as an employee benefit, as "group" health insurance through the parent's workplace, although in some instances families directly purchase "individual" coverage from the insurer. For the most part, both individual and group insurance plans are similarly structured, offering benefits for hospitalization and physicians' services; however, individual coverage is typically much more costly and offers fewer benefits.

Even with seemingly adequate health insurance, many families with children with complex medical conditions find themselves with major financial burdens because of the limitations and terms of coverage. Specific problematic provisions include (1) lack of coverage of preexisting conditions; (2) deductibles, co-insurance, and stop-loss limits; (3) lifetime ceiling on benefits; and (4) depth and breadth of coverage for needed services.

Many private insurance companies deny or restrict coverage of preexisting conditions, health conditions that were known at the time that the insurance went into effect. These limitations are particularly burdensome because they deny (or postpone) coverage to those people who most need it (those *with* health problems) and also force families to pay expensive out-of-pocket costs for needed health care while waiting for coverage. Rather than accept this risk, most families choose to forgo job transfers or other life changes that will affect insurance or coverage. Other families learn about preexisting condition exclusions only after making a job move, too late to avoid the loss of needed health insurance. In recent years, the availability of employer-based health insurance coverage for children with special health needs has eroded in two ways (Rosenbaum, 1988). First, as a cost-cutting measure, many employers have stopped providing health insurance for dependents or offer it only at high cost to the employee, an extra burden for young families with marginal incomes. Second, to save money, employers increasingly change the carrier from whom they purchase medical insurance, and the new insurer may apply a preexisting condition clause, thus removing needed coverage even when the employee has not changed jobs.

The family's out-of-pocket expenses are largely determined by the deductible, co-insurance, and stop-loss provisions of private health insurance. The deductible is the amount the family must pay out-of-pocket before insurance pays for services; co-insurance is the percentage of the provider's bill that the family is expected to pay; stop-loss coverage is the maximum amount that the family will pay before insurance covers all services. Although the cost to families with able-bodied children for these provisions may be substantial but not devastating, the ongoing annual burden of these expenses for a family with a medically complex child can severely undermine the family's financial stability (American Academy of Pediatrics, 1987).

The lifetime ceiling on benefits is a provision of health insurance that families with able-bodied children often ignore but that families with children with complex medical conditions find of major concern. While people in good health may believe that $1 million of health insurance coverage is more than enough to cover any medical need, families with ventilator-dependent or other medically fragile children will attest to its limitations. One family expected that their ventilator-dependent son would use his entire $1 million of coverage before his second birthday, and they were preparing to apply for the Medicaid waiver in their state when we met them.

Although most third-party payers provide adequate coverage for hospitalization and physician services, few insurers offer satisfactory benefits for home care. Policies that provide home-care benefits usually apply many restrictions. In most cases, coverage for home-care services is linked to recent hospitalization; services are provided in lieu of hospitalization; and the recipient of services must be at home or homebound, a limitation rarely applying to children. Implicit in these requirements is the assumption that home care costs the insurer less. In many cases, cost savings must be demonstrated for coverage of home-care services.

Many, but not all, group insurance plans provide coverage for the special home services needed by families of chronically ill children. Fox and Newacheck (1990) documented the breadth and depth of benefits provided by group insurance policies in a survey of 150 employers, of which 140 provided medical insurance coverage to employees. Of the 140 firms offering coverage, 122 (87 percent) provided visiting nurse benefits; 104 (74 percent) covered home health aides; 96 (69 percent) covered home-care services such as occupational, speech, physical, and respiratory therapy and social work, but 75 percent of these firms limited visits. There were 129 firms (92 percent) that covered mental health counseling, but 52 limited the number of sessions per year, and 34 applied other limits; and 72 firms (51 percent) offered individual benefits management. As is evident from these data, the available benefits for home-care services meet the basic needs of most families but are likely to be inadequate in scope and depth to meet the needs of a family with a child with a complex medical condition.

Benefit limitations have a powerful impact on out-of-pocket expenses to families. A child requiring weekly speech therapy and physical therapy (a combined total of 104 sessions annually) will rapidly exhaust coverage when total therapy visits are limited to 60 per year. This family will be responsible for paying for the remaining 44 sessions that are uninsured. An additional burden of 20 percent co-payment requirements, often applied to home-care benefits, imposes further costs. Assuming moderate therapy charges of $50 per session, the family of this child will be responsible for paying 20 percent of the charges for the first 60 sessions and full charges for the 44 remaining sessions. For speech and physical therapies alone, this family will have out-of-pocket costs of $2800. Such expenses are beyond the means of most families.

Other restrictions in coverage for home health care services for children abound. Insurers may cover direct home nursing procedures but will often not reimburse for education about illness or training family caregivers. Likewise, many insurers insist (as they do for adults) that a child must be at home and all services must be provided in the home. This requirement precludes payment by insurance for private-duty nursing at school for a ventilator-dependent child who requires around-the-clock care. Other idiosyncracies of coverage that restrict benefits defy rational explanation but may be explained by an aversion to setting precedent: An insurer was willing to pay for nursing care but was unwilling to pay for a less costly homemaker so that the child's mother, a nurse herself, could have time to provide care.

PREPAID GROUP PRACTICE

Prepaid group practices (such as health maintenance organizations or independent practice associations) are conceptually attractive models for providing care and coverage to children with complex health conditions. These practices agree to provide inpatient and outpatient care and a range of additional services in exchange for a fixed total payment (usually paid monthly). Prepaid practices therefore should have incentives to provide many services (beyond basic hospitalization and physicians' services) that families with medically complex children need—for example, preventive care, preventive mental health services, home care, and care coordination—in order to prevent costly hospitalization.

A survey of prepaid group practices by Fox and colleagues (1990) sheds some light on the adequacy of these organizations in meeting the needs of children with complex medical conditions. In general, prepaid group practices offer very good coverage for acute care services but are less generous in their benefits for chronic care. The use of primary-care physicians as "gate-keepers" who must authorize many services restricts children's access to services such as specialty physicians, hospital outpatient departments, ancillary services (such as occupational, physical, and speech therapies), mental health services, and substance abuse treatment. Additional restrictions on the use of these benefits may be applied through limitations on the number of visits or dollar amount of services that will be covered. Home health benefits are covered by nearly all the plans surveyed, but, again, access is limited by physician referral or other requirements. Case management is usually offered as a limited service but does not include the multidisciplinary, comprehensive focus that families with medically complex children require.

Restrictions on access to services must be traded off against the clear benefits of prepaid group practice enrollment: Families have low out-of-pocket expenses and excellent protection against the catastrophic cost of hospitalization. An additional benefit, not significant to most families with apparently well children but of crucial importance to families with children with complex medical conditions, is that the prepaid group practices in the survey rarely exclude coverage for preexisting conditions.

Unfortunately, there is little conclusive evidence about the actual performance of prepaid group practices in caring for children with complex medical conditions. Some families are very satisfied with the care and services they receive, having learned to "work the system" to get the most from their plans, yet many anecdotes from other families and from providers indicate that prepaid group practices fall short of their potential in meeting families' needs. In particular, access to specialty providers is reported to be restricted, thereby denying children access to needed services; and contrary to the results of the Fox survey, home-care benefits are said to be severely limited and inadequate to meet the needs of medically complex children at home.

TITLE V PROGRAM FOR CHILDREN WITH SPECIAL HEALTH CARE NEEDS

The programs for Children with Special Health Care Needs (CSHCN), formerly the Crippled Children's Service, are operated in the 50 states and the territories as largely independent programs whose policies and procedures are determined at the state level. This independence gives states the freedom to establish eligibility requirements, both financial and medical (that is, some conditions are covered while others are not), and to define the range of covered or provided services. In general, the programs for CSHCN serve low-income children, treating primarily orthopedic and surgical conditions and, to a lesser extent, medical and behavioral problems (Ireys & Eichler, 1988).

While this flexibility allows states to target resources to fill gaps in the health services system, it also creates inequities among states (Ireys, Hauck, & Perrin, 1985). Children with a condition such as severe asthma may receive services in one state but lack coverage in a neighboring state. One state may deny a child eligibility because of excess family income but another may cover the child because of different income standards. Some states may cover primary care for all enrolled children while others may pay only for services related to the specific chronic condition.

In 1989 OBRA changed the allocation of federal funds and the reporting requirements for Title V and CSHCN programs. These regulations require that all states allocate at least 30 percent of the federal block grant to programs for primary and preventive care for children and at least 30 percent to programs for children with special health care needs. Establishing minimum funding levels helps assure that all states provide at least minimal services to all groups targeted by Title V. The new Title V reporting obligations of OBRA 1989 mandate that states report the number of children with chronic illness and their conditions (Fox, 1990).

Inadequate funding limits the ability of CSHCN programs to finance services for children. Nevertheless, these programs can offer many other important benefits. They often provide a focal point in state government to advocate for the special needs of children, and they are in a unique position to promulgate and enforce standards of care. Their influence can extend far beyond the limited funds at their disposal to promote care to children with special medical needs.

THE INDIVIDUALS WITH DISABILITIES EDUCATION ACT (P.L. 94–142 AND ITS REVISIONS)

The Education of the Handicapped Act of 1975 (EHA, or P.L. 94–142) was landmark legislation whose purpose was to "to assure the free appropriate public education of all handicapped children" (U.S. Congress, 1983). This legislation has assured that children with handicaps and other health impairments receive education and additional related services that are necessary for them to benefit from school. Public Law 99–457 extended the provisions of the original Education of the Handicapped Act and provided states with resources to extend services to the population of children up to 3 years of age. This act encouraged early identification and prevention of conditions that might affect a child's long-term ability to be educated. In 1991, the act was revised and renamed the Individuals With Disabilities Education Act (IDEA). An important task in the implementation of IDEA will be the determination of mechanisms to integrate these different public resources in providing services for children with severe illnesses—integrating educational programs and resources with Medicaid and private health insurance programs.

Many children (for example, those who are mentally retarded, learning disabled, and orthopedically impaired) have enormously benefitted from EHA, having suffered from restricted educational opportunities before the law's implementation. The impact of EHA on children with complex chronic conditions has been variable because many such children do not meet eligibility requirements when they are narrowly applied and because states' implementation of the act's provisions have been variable. However, those children with chronic conditions who *are* determined to be eligible under the provisions of this legislation (usually being classified in the "other health impaired" category) have access to an expansive array of services at no cost to the family.

The provisions of P.L. 94–142 entitle eligible children to an education in the least restrictive environment and to services that help the child benefit from his or her education. Many health-related services are included, where those services are determined essential to the child's participation in school. Health-related services can include physical and occupational therapy, speech and language therapy, psychological services, social work, and recreational services. Other services, such as home instruction, medication administration during the school day, and transportation, might also be offered. Access to such services through school can make the difference in a child's remaining current with peers or falling behind in his or her education and socialization (Baird & Ashcroft, 1985).

The number of children served and the spending levels on services under EHA are substantial. During the school year 1985–1986, a total of 50,478 children aged 3 to 21 were served by EHA in the other-health-impaired category; these children represent 1.2 percent of the total of 4,112,729 youngsters served by EHA. During 1984–85, a total of 29,365 children in the other-health-impaired category received physical therapy, 9539 received occupational therapy, 11,798 received speech and language services, 14,936 had psychological counseling, and 25,478 received transportation. Although the percentage of children in the other-health-impaired category who receive these services is high, they represent a small percent of the totals; during 1984–1985, a total of 128,574 children received physical therapy; 139,961 got occupational therapy; and 665,555 received speech and language services; 772,144 children received psychological services, and 1,006,726 had special transportation. Altogether federal, state, and local authorities spent in 1985–1986 approximately $3 billion for all related services under EHA (U.S. Department of Education, 1987; U.S. Department of Education, 1990).

THE UNINSURED AND UNDERINSURED

The uninsured and underinsured are two groups whom the private and public health care financing systems have failed. Estimates of the size of these groups vary with each survey and definition, but they represent many millions of people, and children are disproportionately included in their ranks (American Academy of Pediatrics, 1987). Of the estimated 37 million Americans without health insurance coverage as of 1986 (Wilensky, 1988), over 12 million are children under age 18 (McManus & Greaney, 1988). Most uninsured children live in families in which at least one parent is employed. Over half these uninsured youngsters live in households in which at least one parent worked full-time throughout the year. A third of uninsured children live in families in which the head works part-time or part of the year. Only 12 percent of uninsured children live in families whose parents are unemployed (McManus, 1989).

The number of underinsured people depends on the definition of underinsurance that is selected. By one definition of underinsurance, an estimated 23.3 percent of children are underinsured (5.9 percent are underinsured according to the definition, 8.4 percent are uninsured all year, and 9.0 percent are uninsured part of the year) (Farley, 1985). But, because of the enormous needs, nearly all families with medically complex children feel that they are underinsured.

Tackling the problems of the uninsured and the underinsured involves two separate issues. The problem for the *uninsured* centers on gaining access to appropriate, affordable health insurance. For the *underinsured,* the problem reflects a need to gain ongoing coverage with sufficient depth and breadth to protect the family from catastrophe. Meeting the needs of underinsured and uninsured children with severe illnesses will require offering coverage that has the following characteristics: no limitations on coverage for preexisting conditions; stable coverage that does not change with parental income, employment, and residence; low stop-loss coverage limits; and broad benefits that include extensive home-care services. The several options offered in recent years for addressing the needs of the uninsured include Medicaid expansions; Medicaid buy-in programs; and state-mandated, employer-paid insurance with state-provided coverage for the unemployed.

Proposals for high-risk pools and for catastrophic insurance are particularly relevant to families with uninsured children with chronic medical problems. States, through their regulation of insurance, can require health care insurers to form high-risk pools to provide health insurance to uninsurable people, those who are otherwise unable to purchase insurance through regular sources. States usually subsidize pools, either by subsidizing sliding fee scales to permit lower-income families to enroll or by tax credits for the participating insurers. Individuals usually become eligible to purchase high-risk insurance by documenting that they have been denied comparable coverage from the regular private insurance system for health reasons. Eligible families can then purchase insurance for their children from the pool at a rate varying from 125 to 400 percent (limit set by the state) of the rate for comparable coverage for an *individual* policy. These higher insurance rates, combined with significant out-of-pocket expenses from high deductibles and co-insurance, delays in coverage for preexisting conditions, and family responsibility for the many noncovered services (typically including home health care), make coverage through high-risk pools unaffordable and impractical for most families. Premiums alone can be sufficiently expensive that only high-income families can afford them. Indeed, only 1 to 2 percent of eligible children have joined high-risk pools where they exist (Fox, 1984; Fox et al., 1987). In the 15 states that have risk-pool arrangements, only 24,355 people of all ages had enrolled through 1987; thus, high-risk pools have only minimally penetrated their intended market of uninsurable clients (Laudicina, 1988).

The Tennessee high-risk pool illustrates the major provisions of this health care financing option. Eligibility for high-risk insurance requires Tennessee residents to document that either they have been rejected for similar health insurance coverage, their health care benefits have been reduced or a medical condition has been excluded, or their health insurance premiums have been increased above the rates charged by the pool. Premiums depend on location of residence, age, sex, and the deductible level ($500 or $2000). As of July 1987, for a child under 18 years old living in Nashville, the annual premium for the $500 deductible plan was $550.23. With this deductible plan, the family's maximum out-of-pocket expenses for covered services (not including the premium itself) will be $1500. However, these expenses do not include any extra payment to providers in excess of the "usual and customary" fees reimbursed by the pool. Benefits are generally comparable to those of many basic policies; home health care benefits are limited to $40 per visit and 270 visits per year. The plan has a lifetime maximum benefit of $500,000. Significantly, coverage excludes preexisting conditions for the first six months that the policy is in effect. While this coverage offers a family some protection from burdensome medical expenses, its high cost for basic benefits limits its attraction to families and makes it unaffordable to all but the most financially secure.

High-risk pools could serve a large number of children who have severe health impairments if their costs to families were much lower and if the benefits more directly addressed the needs of these children and their families. In their current form they represent a state subsidy for relatively high-income families, those who can afford the hefty premiums. Making high-risk pools applicable to home care for larger numbers of children will require major changes in the structure of high-risk-pool insurance and major new funding.

Catastrophic health insurance programs have been designed to address some problems of underinsurance (Weeks, 1985). Essentially a reinsurance program for times when "ordinary" insurance is insufficient, catastrophic coverage provides for individuals who have incurred huge medical bills in a short time. Catastrophic health insurance best meets the needs of people who experience sudden medical problems with associated great expense. Given the pattern of expenses experienced by most children with complex medical conditions—

high expenses each year, rarely reaching catastrophic proportions in a single year—few families become eligible for coverage under these programs, even though the *long-term* costs can be catastrophic. Those families who do qualify receive benefits only for a defined time period and lose benefits when this period expires. Families may become eligible again for catastrophic insurance benefits after they again incur large medical bills. This on/off pattern of coverage repeats the experience of many children on Medicaid whose care suffers from interruption of eligibility. Beyond these limitations, catastrophic insurance often excludes benefits for home care and other services needed by severely ill youngsters. Although catastrophic health insurance may rescue a family from overwhelming debt from medical care, it is not designed or intended to provide the ongoing, basic health care benefits that severely ill children need.

SUMMARY AND IMPLICATIONS

Most children requiring home care do have fairly extensive insurance coverage for many of their expenses. But gaps in coverage, both from noncovered services and from times when coverage is not in effect, leave families at risk for unaffordable medical expenses. And the incentives are often wrong, encouraging hospitalization and institutional care. Families have had to fight long and arduous battles to make the system provide humane, family-centered, and home-based care.

The current system of health insurance, tied largely to steady employment at well-paying jobs or to poverty, creates an environment in which parents are hostages to the status quo: Parents living in poverty cannot afford to earn additional income and risk losing Medicaid benefits, whereas middle-income parents cannot afford to change jobs and risk losing current employer-based insurance coverage.

To finance health services, the nation needs a system of health insurance with national standards, assuring an adequate level of care for all children. Such a system would provide the same basic benefits to children regardless of the parents' economic status or place of residence. However, universal health insurance alone will not meet the needs of children with severe illnesses. The extra financial burdens their families carry merit additional benefits, such as cash payments through SSI or tax breaks. Health insurance and extra financial benefits would help offset parents' stress from economic worries and allow them to focus on their top priority—taking care of their children with special health needs.

7

Recommendations

PRINCIPLES

Three main principles guide our recommendations for public policy in home and community care for children with special health needs. These principles are based on our respect for the dedication and accomplishments of parents and families in the face of many obstacles, and they reflect themes that persist throughout our investigation. Families find many effective services and committed professionals but also frequent limitations in family service and support systems. The three principles, explored further in the next sections, are: (1) Families must have the central role in guiding the care for their children; (2) the base of services must be broad and flexible, reflecting family needs that change over time; and (3) children in home care must be integrated into the fabric of their communities.

Centrality of Families

Families must be allowed to determine the course of care for their children. To the extent possible, they should direct which services will be provided, who will provide them, and the means by which services will be provided. Implicit in this statement is a broad focus on the child in a family and community context rather than a narrow perspective on the treatment of a child's health problem. Policies should ensure the empowerment of families so that they can direct with confidence the programs that best nurture the growth and development of their children. Families should be encouraged to claim from the system the services that they believe their children need, and they should be secure enough to deal with the variety of providers and vendors who may offer services to their children. Families also need access to services to help other family members whose lives are affected by home care, services such as counseling and respite. Achieving these goals requires that families acquire new knowledge and skills in providing care and in managing complex systems of care, and families may find these tasks daunting. Providers too must work hard to help families achieve this knowledge and skill. Families will need information, education, and careful explanations of options to make informed decisions even though the outcomes of many choices may be uncertain.

Flexibility and Breadth of Services

Families need access to a flexible and broad range of services. Flexibility is required because families' needs change over time as the child and family grow and develop. Breadth of services is necessary because children's conditions and family life are multifaceted. Families need access to a continuum of services—specialized inpatient services; respite and day-care services; home-, school-, and community-based treatment; and support services. Providers should recognize that children and their families may require different services along this continuum at different times during children's development. For instance, families in the early days of home care may greatly value in-home nursing services but may wish, at a later time, to assume more direct care responsibility for themselves, substituting respite opportunities for nursing services. Flexibility in meeting families' needs is a cornerstone to the provision of adequate home care.

Integration into Communities

Families and children in home care need to be integrated into the fabric of their communities. Policies and programs should encourage this integration. The issue here goes well beyond the provision of medical and health services. The majority of children requiring home care can participate in usual activities of other children, especially school. Children and families deserve access to all community services, including day care, recreation, community-based health care, preschool education, and schooling in the least restrictive environment.

A RATIONALE FOR ACTION: VIEWING THE APPROACHES

Why should public policies and programs respond to the home-care needs of severely ill children and their families? It could be argued that relatively few youngsters have a severe health impairment that requires home-based services and that those few families facing these problems must themselves arrange and provide for home- and community-based services. With many American children lacking access to basic health services, why should public policy address the problem of severely ill children? At times, as we have shown, public programs provide some help through Medicaid or model waiver programs, Title V programs for Children with Special Health Care Needs, or SSI. If families currently obtain most of the services they need, is further public attention warranted?

Public attitudes and policies in the United States lean toward notions of self-reliance and of individual and family responsibility, rather than societal responsibility, for the care of individuals with disability. The problems of a child with a severe long-term illness are viewed mainly as a family concern, with little support from the society at large, yet there are strong arguments for strengthening society's concerns for families with children with severe illnesses. These arguments can be based on humanitarian, prudential, utilitarian, and equity reasons.

On purely humanitarian grounds, all children merit access to services that will improve their health status. Further, the nature of severe illness is such that any family may be affected, usually unexpectedly. Thus, it may be prudent to have services available in the case that any of us may face this special need (Kopelman, 1985). Utilitarian concepts argue that the changing demography of society, with increasing numbers of elderly, creates a pressing need that every child be adequately prepared to be economically productive and provide resources to support society in general (Committee for Economic Development, 1987). Insofar as most children with severe illnesses survive to adulthood and can become productive members of society, the utilitarian notion argues for reasonable investments during the lifetime of these individuals to maximize their later contributions to society. In general, equal access to a reasonable level of health is a notion with which many people can agree; means of defining equity and assuring equitable access may be more controversial (Outka, 1975). The equity argument suggests that health services that may prevent or diminish health disability and that are available to anyone should be available to everyone.

European nations have a different notion of responsibility for long-term care and the care of people with disability. In general, Europeans view the responsibility as one that should be shared between society and the family rather than borne mainly by the family with little community help. In England, social security benefits are available for children with special health needs and their families (Goodwin, 1990). Children who require significant in-home care because of disability receive government payments, and a higher payment is made for youngsters with disability who need nighttime as well as daytime care. Furthermore, the parents receive an additional allowance if they themselves provide care for their children. Children over age 5 who are unable to walk receive a mobility allowance. These payments, like payments in other

European countries, are made to all families affected, regardless of income. A similarly broad view of the social contract with families would help American children function more effectively over time.

What policy efforts may then aid American children with severe illnesses and their families? Several approaches could be considered for responding to the needs of these families. Our view, as we shall describe later in this chapter, argues for a comprehensive three-pronged approach: (1) a universal health care effort providing basic services to all people, (2) additional support for the organization and maintenance of systems of care for children with special health needs, and (3) specific financial benefits to support families. Yet other approaches, some incorporating just one of the three elements proposed here and others quite different, are possible. These other approaches include: (1) withholding public resources for the specialized care of children with severe illness until a satisfactory base of services is available to all children (the "greatest good" approach) or (2) maintaining the current level of investment in these children without change (the "status quo" approach).

Public priorities could require distributing limited resources by building a floor of basic health service coverage for all youngsters including those with serious illnesses. This "greatest good" approach might call for redistributing current funding for health services for disabled children to all children through a universal health insurance scheme, with a narrow benefit package. Children with disabilities are at especially high risk of lacking insurance (Butler et al., 1985a), although some, especially those with severe disabling conditions, at least gain access to Medicaid through the Supplemental Security Income program (Perrin & Stein, 1991). Providing entitlement to basic health services for all children would greatly benefit children with severe health conditions. Nevertheless, improving access to basic health insurance will not address adequately the broad and complex needs of children with severe illness and their families. Health insurance can support traditional medical and surgical services and some preventive services, but it offers little support for home- and community-based care or adherence to the principles of families' central role, broad and flexible services, and the integration of children into their communities.

The risks of this greatest good approach should not be minimized. Underlying this approach, at least in part, is the erroneous notion that increasing access of children and families to preventive and primary health care will significantly decrease the number of children born with severe illness and thereby decrease the number of children who require complex long-term health and related services. This notion reflects a belief that the incidence of many disabling conditions can be reduced through these services. Yet, a careful review of the causes of the many forms of severe illness in childhood indicates that a minority can be prevented by currently known preventive and primary health services (Holtzman & Richmond, 1985). Thus the approach of allocating more resources to preventive and primary health care services will not decrease in a major way the frequency of severe illnesses among children. For the foreseeable future, there will be a significant population of severely ill children, just as there will be a significant and increasing population of seriously ill older people.

The 1991 Institute of Medicine (IOM) report on the prevention of disability in America (Institute of Medicine, 1991) distinguished between the prevention of disabling conditions and the prevention of the psychosocial and economic consequences of disabling conditions already present. Although the IOM noted progress in the prevention of certain disabling health conditions, the report also stressed opportunities to diminish the impact of a health condition on the ability to work and to enjoy a reasonable quality of life.

Maintaining the current system represents a status quo approach. Current efforts emphasize maintaining medical stability, not enhancing development. This approach exacerbates the fragmentation of services, leaves many needs of families unmet, and limits the potential contribution of many children and families. A version of this approach includes redistribution of resources to improve efficiency in the system. Current child health expenditures in the United States average over $700 per child per year, from both public and private sources. Coordination of these expenditures, with less waste, could improve health care for all children.

Cost containment has motivated health policy in the past decade (Sloan, Blumstein, & Perrin, 1988). Although greater efficiency in the use of health resources will help to restrain expenditures, any programs for people with disability, and especially severe disability, will require major investments at least in the short run. Disability is expensive for families and society, as most industrialized countries recognize. The most effective way to achieve savings in the short run would be to curtail all programs that support children with severe health conditions, including medical and surgical care, yet this policy would lead to higher death rates and would make survivors more dependent on public institutions in their later years. This approach is unlikely to be chosen by parents, professionals, or policymakers.

The main rationale for why public policy should address the problem of seriously ill children and their families is that a nation as wealthy as the United States cannot justify ignoring the service needs of a segment of its population. Even with universal access to effective preventive and primary health care services, children and families will continue to face severe illnesses, and their needs will be best met through the three-pronged approach that we describe below.

THE ELEMENTS OF ACTION

Empowering families and improving the lives of severely ill children demand attention in three areas: organization and provision of services; determination and improvement of quality; and financial support of families. Policy is often implemented in piecemeal fashion, with one element or another rather than with a comprehensive plan. We believe, however, that all three elements are necessary if the nation intends to maximize the potential of these children. The *financial* support for these efforts in turn includes four facets: direct financial support for families; universal access to basic health services; funding for special benefits for children with severe illnesses and their families; and support for the organization of special systems of care for these children.

The Organization and Provision of Services

Our observations have led us to conclude that families need services in five broad areas: in-home direct care services; services that promote integration into the community; services to support families; services on a continuum from hospital to home to community and including respite care; and case management or care coordination. While these areas are not entirely distinct, they incorporate approaches that are needed by all families who face the challenge of home-based care.

In-home Direct Care Services

In-home direct care includes a variety of services—private-duty nursing with extensive hours of care for children with the most complex conditions (typically, ventilator-dependent); episodic home health nursing; physical, occupational, or other therapies; home health aides; homemakers; babysitters; and home visitors. As exemplified in several of the cases cited in earlier chapters, flexibility should be the hallmark of in-home services. Although third-party payers may rigidly limit the type of in-home nursing services, families often need a more comprehensive and flexible array of services including homemaker, direct nursing, other associated direct therapies such as respiratory therapy and nutrition, and skilled babysitting.

We recommend the expansion of child-oriented home-health care programs supported by flexible home-care benefits by public and private third-party payers. The current organization of in-home services leaves most programs ill-equipped to provide the services that children and families need. Because of reimbursement requirements and constraints, most nursing agencies emphasize health care *procedures* in the home and neglect issues of family empowerment and care coordination. The emphasis on procedures neglects the help

desired by families—education about illness and its treatment, child development, encouragement of family competence in caretaking, and homemaker
services. Home nursing agencies will need organizational reorientation and
financial incentives to offer to non-procedurally oriented services.

Nurses are mainly, although not exclusively, well trained to provide services to these children and families, yet nursing home health agencies are not
the only organizations that should be encouraged to expand their child-
oriented home-care efforts. Some nursing agencies may have difficulty expanding from providing direct nursing services to offering broader home-care
services including education, child development, and specialized therapies,
especially in a developmentally appropriate way for young children. Other
organizations may have the broader vision necessary to provide direct in-home
services successfully. Many of the functions of public health nursing fit well
with the needs of families providing care to children at home. These functions
include home and family assessment, knowledge of and referral to community
resources, and family education. Integration of public health nursing functions
in some communities with clinical nursing in the home setting may improve
quality.

Integration into the Community

Community integration is an additional goal not only for children with severe
health conditions but also their families. Children merit access to both specialized and regular community services such as libraries, clubs, recreation,
day care, schools, public transportation, shopping malls, and all other aspects
of community life that are part of the daily routine of other families. Although
typically considered recipients only of specialized services, most children with
complex medical conditions grow and continue to live in their own communities. To "normalize" their growth and development, they need the opportunity to go to school, to use all the regular services, and to participate in
activities available to other youngsters.

Most severely ill children can become productive members of society.
Whether a child will do well and prosper is difficult to determine in the short
term or in the individual case; however, early intervention to prevent or
diminish disability helps make these youngsters become more productive
members of society and less dependent over time on public institutions. The
model of early intervention for very young children with developmental disabilities may be appropriate as well for children with long-term illnesses or
significant need for home care. When early intervention services are organized
properly they provide a flexible model that addresses health, early childhood
education, and social concerns, as well as family support and education
(Meisels & Shonkoff, 1990). Analysis of the Infant Health and Development

Program, a carefully controlled experiment, demonstrated impressive improvements among children at high risk of developing problems in their social and intellectual functioning (Infant Health and Development Program, 1990).

Expanding this model of community intervention to children with complex long-term illnesses and, where appropriate, to children who are older than those currently involved in most early intervention programs may be a promising way to maximize children's developmental progress. Similarly, for older youngsters, direct attention to vocational preparation especially in the adolescent years can maximize their functioning (Hippolitus, 1985), and recent evidence supports the importance of beginning vocational planning by early adolescence. More flexibility in the way that services for these children are funded, along with additional support for unmet needs, will help families raise offspring who are more capable of joining adult society.

A central part of optimal community integration is that the child be educated in the least restrictive environment. A child who is ventilator-dependent will likely need specialized in-school health services and the ability to have equipment at hand, but that child may not require special education services in order to learn well. As shown in Chapter 3, schools must use flexible definitions of special needs in providing appropriate health-related services to assure the least restrictive environment for children with severe illnesses.

Family Support Services
Caring for a child with a complex medical condition requires addressing not only the health needs and social development of the child but also the concerns of all family members. Just as a child's requirements change over time, so do the family's. As needs evolve, families require access to a wide range of support services: family counseling (including genetic counseling when appropriate), support groups, babysitting, day care, respite, and alternative placement.

Babysitting and day care offer frequent, short-term breaks from the pressures of ongoing responsibility for the care of a medically complex child and also afford parents an opportunity to work at paid employment, thereby maintaining valuable health care benefits. Unfortunately, these services are difficult for families to find, and if available at all, they are costly. Babysitting by extended family members, a valuable resource for many, is rarely available because family members often fear assuming responsibility for the care of these children. Similarly, few day-care centers are staffed to provide safe care to a child with special health needs. A few specialized day-care programs for medically fragile children have demonstrated the viability of such services. As described in Chapter 3, the Prescribed Pediatric Extended Care program in Tampa, Florida, is a day-care program for children with severe health impairments that meets criteria for reimbursement as a medical service by third-party payers. Although offering no respite services on weekends, the program allows families to pursue other daily activities. Specialized, developmental day-care programs, such as Handicare in Iowa City, also nurture the growth of the child and help to make family life more normal.

Respite care merits special attention. Parents talk frequently about the lack of opportunity to have a break from child care, yet evidence, especially from families in England with children with developmental disabilities, strongly supports the notion that effective respite programs decrease the likelihood of long-term institutionalization of children (Brimblecombe, 1974). Respite improves families' capacities to care for their own children. Although some may question whether respite care fits a category of health services, clear distinctions for these children are difficult. Unfortunately, few respite programs exist, and, to compensate for the gaps in services, families place children in acute-care hospitals or arrange around-the-clock private-duty nursing to take vacations and other breaks in caretaking. Acknowledging the importance of respite care and expanding the system's capacity to provide it are important priorities.

Some families need alternative placements for the care of their children. The viewpoints of biologic parents of children with complex medical conditions who provide care for their children at home dominate this study. Most of these parents believe that their medically impaired children, like able-bodied children, belong at home and that society should provide the support to make this possible. They believe that just as society would never ask the parents of an apparently able-bodied newborn, ''Do you want to bring this infant home from the hospital?,'' they too should not be asked such a question. They view as a foregone conclusion that all parents want to and will bring their children home. Nevertheless, it is clear that some biologic parents are unable, because of their own health status or household resources, to bring these youngsters home. Other parents may have become exhausted by the extensive demands of home care and are no longer able to carry on, and some parents may be unwilling to attempt the effort.

The prevailing assumption that medically complex children must go home to their biologic parents may not fit all children. These youngsters should not languish in hospitals when parents are unable to bring them home. Just as alternative homes are found for able-bodied children whose parents are unable to care for them, alternative settings for raising medically complex children of these families must be identified. While every effort must be made to encourage and to support parents in home care, such care is beyond the ability of some families. In light of the demands of home care for a chronically ill child, it seems likely that neither the child nor the rest of the family will likely do well if home care is imposed on unwilling parents.

If families decide against home care, they leave the way open to consideration of other placements such as foster care, adoption, or residential programs, and in some few situations to continued institutional care in a chronic care or other facility. A few alternatives to home care are institutional; most are community-based and aim to integrate severely health-impaired children into services for other children. Some services should be ongoing and continuous; others are needed by families when their capacity to provide home care is temporarily exhausted. In either case, family members need flexibility to select the appropriate care setting for their child as both the child's and family's needs change.

Recent efforts to develop specialized foster care programs for severely ill children are particularly promising (Gurdin & Anderson, 1991; Prybyl & Prybyl, 1991). Here the special issues of caring for these children in homes and communities are partly addressed through specialized training of foster parents and recruiting parents with relevant professional experience (e.g., nursing).

Continuum of Health and Medical Services

Children with chronic and complex medical conditions need access to a broad range of health and medical services. While we have been impressed that most children and families seem able to obtain tertiary medical services, we have been equally concerned about the apparent dearth of community-based primary care for medically involved children. This gap forces families to continue the costly and inefficient practice of using tertiary-care resources for primary care.

Ideally, multidisciplinary teams, with the family having a central role in all activities, should be the organizational model for services. The needs of families transcend the efforts of practitioners of any single discipline— medicine, nursing, social work, and others. Families may need only one or two different services at any time, but communities will be well served by a variety of professionals working together with families. Successful model programs recognize that family needs are complex and demand careful teamwork, with central roles for families and nurses. And although these models may have nurses as the primary professionals, effective programs tend to define direct nursing care and procedures as a means of establishing relationships with the child and family rather than an end in itself. The objective is the strengthening of the capacity of families to take charge of their own lives.

How best to organize multidisciplinary services varies from one part of the country to another. We propose a system of community-based services in all parts of the nation in which resources are integrated at the community level so as to assure families access to the broad range of home- and community-based services that they need. In each community, some agency must provide the lead for the integration of services, but the great differences among communities call for a pluralistic system rather than a uniform one. Integrated services could be based around schools, neighborhood health centers, regional maternal and child health clinics, community hospitals, public health departments especially in rural areas, area education programs as in Iowa, or specialty care hospitals.

Pivotal program characteristics include the ability to provide a broad array of services at the community level, to monitor and improve quality, to assure the development and monitoring of individual family service plans, and to assure the coordination of services. Programs must be culturally appropriate, taking into account household social and environmental circumstances and the values of caretakers and communities. Programs should have active involvement of families in program management and policy development. Guidelines specifying program characteristics should direct public funding in support of community-based, integrated service programs. Most European countries provide a model for such community efforts through some form of community-based preventive care program (Child Health in 1990). In England, the Health Visitor program has responsibility to identify children with special health needs, assure adequate evaluation, and help families integrate services at the community level. In Norway, community health centers serve a similar purpose. Regional psychoeducational centers in France help assure coordination between mental health and educational services for children with severe chronic illnesses and their families Although European programs provide different degrees of attention to the problems of children with long-term health conditions, they all have a mechanism for integrating services at the community level.

States require a mechanism both to support the development and maintenance of these community-based programs and to assure effective regionalized activities for those times when a child needs very specialized services away from the home community. Each state must have a lead agency providing this direction. Similar to development of programs through Public Law 99–457, appropriate state agencies include health departments, special education programs, and offices for children. Given the health-related aspects of the severe illnesses of childhood, the state Maternal and Child Health Program should have a central role even if it is not the lead agency. The 1989 revision of the Maternal and Child Health Block Grant requires state Title V Services to Children with Special Health Needs programs to give leadership in developing family-centered, community-based systems of care. Furthermore, the National Health Promotion and Disease Prevention Objectives (U.S. Department of Health and Human Services, 1990, Objective 17.20) call for the development in all 50 states of service systems for children with or at risk of chronic and disabling conditions. Coordination of the organizational efforts of the state maternal and child health program, the financing activities of Medicaid and the SSI program, and public education efforts (especially through Public Laws 99–142 and 99–457) is essential to building comprehensive systems of care. The state agency should assure access for all families to integrated programs in their communities, help to initiate and maintain these programs, define standards and monitor performance, provide needed continuing education, and serve as the main public voice in assuring such programs.

Coordination of Care

Families facing a multitude of services and providers need help with care coordination and case management. In most instances, families come to provide their own care coordination effectively as they build their own skills. Yet, especially in the first months of caring for a severely ill child at home, many families benefit from help with the coordination of care from a person outside the family. Family needs shift over time, and our discussions with care coordinators and families suggest that intensive care coordination is rarely needed for longer than 12 to 18 months, with most coordination provided adequately thereafter by families themselves. However, there are times of transition, such as school entry, early adolescence, or aging out of certain programs and services, that may require another period of intense care coordination. The metaphor of the boiling pot of water applies to the need for care coordination. Just as intense heat is required to bring the pot to a boil, but low heat thereafter keeps it simmering, so families' need for intensive services in the early stages diminishes as families learn to take charge.

Most existing model programs employ nurses as care coordinators, although a few programs use personnel with education or social work backgrounds or lay counselors. Important characteristics of care coordinators are flexibility, advocacy, patience, concern and respect for individuals, and decisiveness. Because nurses often have these characteristics and because many needed services are health related, nurses often perform well as coordinators of care. Still, we propose a system that allows flexibility in the determination of who coordinates care. We judge that it is more important to define the parameters of care coordination and management, to see that these responsibilities are carried out, and to see that these services receive equitable reimbursement than it is to specify the profession that receives the assignment. Effective coordination requires a commitment of time and resources often as substantial as the commitment of resources to more traditional health and medical services.

The major elements of care coordination include advocacy for the needs of children and families, aid in deciding among conflicting treatments and priorities, education and information about illness, treatment, and choices, and help with access to services. The care coordinator or manager, whether a member of the family or not, serves mainly as an advocate and extension of the family, assuring the family's access to regular and specialized services. As household needs and abilities change, the family should be able to renegotiate coordination arrangements.

A general physician in the community can help the care coordinator with problems in working with medical services. Community care coordination, however, is broader than coordination of medical services and links the family with the school system and other community services, assures communication with specialty services, and helps families integrate these services into a coherent whole. With this support, community physicians can provide primary medical services to children with severe illnesses and leave many complicated issues of identifying and arranging other services to a care coordinator.

Assuring Quality

How to improve the quality of home-based services is a complex issue. Little supervision is available to nurses working in homes. Because families depend on the availability of nursing services, they may hesitate to question the ability of staff or to complain about services. Although quality issues are difficult to address where services are provided in isolated settings and with little peer or supervisory contact, our visits with families confirmed that quality is of utmost importance.

Quality improvement requires attention to structure, process, and outcome. Key structural items are standards for both personnel and programs. Personnel standards include requirements for training and experience, supervision, and performance. Standards for programs include such issues as the breadth of personnel, sufficient and appropriately maintained equipment, a comprehensive and community-based program model, and methods to assure monitoring. The multidisciplinary nature of the program and its links with community services as well as specialty medical and surgical care should be specified. Mechanisms for incorporating families into decision making should be made clear.

The central process for assuring quality is the individual family service plan. The plan should be developed by the multidisciplinary community-based team, with the active participation and agreement of the family. Plans should set goals for both child and family, indicate when these goals should be achieved, and determine who will be responsible for achieving them. Finally, the plan should state the means for monitoring achievement of the goals and for revising the plan periodically.

The increasing emphasis on measuring outcomes of health care will improve the evaluation of interventions provided to families of children with severe illnesses. Many home-care interventions, such as nursing services, the provision of ancillary therapies, different forms of care coordination, and methods to improve integration of the family into the community, are areas where careful evaluation of effects of interventions on desired outcomes will be beneficial. Such studies have received scant funding and attention. We recommend the development of a comprehensive and coordinated program of research to investigate these questions, recognizing that sizable financial support will be required. Careful epidemiologic work to determine ways of preventing the secondary consequences of severe illness could be carried out by the Centers for Disease Control, an arm of the U.S. Department of Health and Human Services. The Agency for Health Care Policy and Research, another federal health unit, should also stimulate a research program to study the effectiveness of interventions.

Efforts to assure quality will require regulatory mechanisms. Regulation in general and in health care specifically has been viewed unfavorably in the past decade because of the perception that regulation interferes with market forces (Blumstein, 1988), yet the failure of demand to stimulate a supply of services at the community level for severely ill children and their families represents market failure rather than lack of need. Most communities offer few options and limited choices, mainly because the relative rarity of these conditions results in limited demand for services; and families often lack satisfactory information with which to make important choices. Here, regulatory mechanisms will help assure quality services and programs. We recommend the development of regulatory bodies comprised of professionals, parents, and young adults with health disability, with responsibilities to examine reimbursement policies, determine standards for personnel and programs, and review and monitor outcomes of care. Third-party payers (or their designees, such as Title V programs) should take into account the findings of these boards in determining their payment policies. States should have this regulatory authority, within national guidelines. The lead state agency, often the Title V program, should coordinate closely with the regulatory body and should have main responsibilities for developing state policies for systems development, establishing minimum standards, and evaluating service systems.

Families and caregivers may disagree on what constitutes quality care.

There is more to quality than the technical ability to get the job done, and the family is in the best position to assess the performance of what is happening in the home. Given the difficulty of assessing the quality of health care providers, services, and programs, families may seek help from program personnel or from regulatory bodies, but they should have the central role in determining what outcomes are important for them and their child and whether those outcomes are being achieved. Where families and other caregivers disagree, there must be recourse to a means of reconciling differing views of quality of care and resolving disagreements in ways that help families.

Financing the Care of Children with Severe Illnesses

Financial support for families whose children have severe illnesses should include: (1) direct financial subsidy to families, (2) universal coverage of basic health care for all children, (3) support for specific benefits for children with long-term illnesses, and (4) adequate financing for the organization of programs for children with special health needs.

Direct Support of Families

A child with a significant long-term health condition creates special financial needs for a family, regardless of the family's social or financial situation. In many European countries this need is recognized through the provision of direct financial benefits to families whose children have significant health disability. In Scandinavian countries it is part of the social contract that families raising a severely ill child receive direct financial subsidy from the government to meet these additional burdens (Lie, 1990). European programs apply no means tests, recognizing that the financial burdens affect all families, regardless of income.

As an issue of family rights, we propose a similar program of public support through direct financial aid to families who have a severely ill child. The option might be considered an expanded Supplemental Security Income (SSI) program for disabled children, except that it carries no means test. This recommendation calls for a broad and generic definition of disability based on functional assessment rather than diagnostic labels, thereby including children with a wide variety of health conditions. Implementation would be through direct cash payments, much like the current SSI program. A cash support system allows families to choose among the services available, from in-home nursing to homemaking to respite services, thereby encouraging and allowing families to set their own priorities. Such systems assume that either essential services currently exist and families simply need the resources to purchase them or that a new financial support program will produce sufficient demand to develop needed services. We judge that family financing, although necessary, is insufficient to assure the availability of needed services of high quality.

Financing Services and Programs

How might additional needed services and programs best be financed? We recommend three additional areas to supplement the direct financial support of families: universal health insurance to support most direct medical services; specific, directly financed health benefits for severely ill children; and additional resources to develop and maintain adequate regionalized systems of care to provide community-based services for severely ill children and their families.

Much recent discussion has focused on means of assuring that every American has access to a basic minimum of health services through a universal health insurance program. Some proposals focus on certain populations, such as children and pregnant women; others cover all Americans (Kinzer, 1990). Some call for greater public financing; others mandate that employers pay for worker and dependent health coverage. Children are disproportionately overrepresented among the uninsured; and those children with chronic illnesses are even more likely to lack adequate basic health coverage (Butler et al., 1985a). Given that basic coverage is essential for all children, we recommend that basic health, medical, and related services be covered and provided through a universal health insurance program. Whether financing comes from public or private sources is less important for children than assuring universal eligibility for health insurance.

Insurance programs to meet the needs of mothers and children must offer different benefits from those necessary for health care for employed adults. Preventive care services are especially important for children and include both common preventive services such as immunizations or screening for lead poisoning or anemia, and also preventive mental health care and services to help parents prevent a child's health problem from interfering with optimal growth and development. Thus a universal health access program should be able to provide specific benefits appropriate to children's needs.

Still, families with children with severe illnesses have further service needs that are unlikely to be covered by traditional basic health insurance programs. Some needed services fall into a category of direct care services, such as in-home nursing or specialized homemaker services; respite and hospice care; equipment; specialized transportation; or coordination of care. Some services may be available through the "basic" insurance program, but many will require a supplemental benefit package that should be available to families whose children meet a broad and generic definition of severe chronic illness. Although these benefits could be financed in a generally available universal insurance program, they presumably will not be available to all families, but rather just to those meeting specific eligibility criteria. Eligibility could be determined in the same fashion as used to determine eligibility for the direct family financial benefit. Despite concerns that the aggregate costs of this broader benefit will be high, the numbers of children and families requiring it represent a small percentage of families, and the mechanisms of determining eligibility should target the benefit to those families who clearly need it.

Health insurance will not, in and of itself, assure the availability of many services needed by families. The development of systems of care based on the principles that introduce this chapter requires additional funding. Here, the state lead agency should have a major role, assessing unmet community needs, nurturing the growth of programs that meet these needs, assuring adequate funding and monitoring of programs, and assuring the development of an adequate structure in which needed services can be delivered. Insurance mechanisms, even with specialized home or long-term benefits, are targeted primarily to the individual or the family. Development of effective community-based preventive programs or regionalized systems of care is unlikely when financing is limited to insurance mechanisms. Furthermore, the many related issues of developing standards, monitoring child health and program outcomes within a state, and providing community and professional education are all additional efforts that insurance programs alone will hardly support. Much of this funding should derive from direct support of state agency activities in these areas; other support should come through direct funding of community agencies or regional programs that assure the development of accessible, family-centered systems of care.

SUMMARY

Three main principles must guide policy and programs for home and community care for children with complex long-term illnesses: self-determination by families; a broad and flexible base of services; and the integration of children into their own communities. Meeting these principles will require a social commitment to supporting families' care of children with severe illnesses. The concept of home- and community-based services should be broad enough to include in-home direct care services, services that promote integration into the community, a broad continuum of services, and care coordination. Respite care is of special importance to these families. Ensuring quality will require the development of broad systems to provide oversight of childhood home care and that have authority to set standards, monitor outcomes, and affect change where needed. Families must have a central role in all of these processes.

Finally, the financial support for childhood home care will be best met through a four-part effort: These parts include direct financial subsidy to families whose children have major health problems; universal health care coverage for all Americans; specific benefits for children with special health needs; and adequate resources to develop and maintain systems of care that provide regionalized and community-based services for severely ill children and their families. The investment of concern and dollars will result in a more vibrant and effective group of young children entering adulthood as members of American society.

References

Adam, H. M. (1989). "Pediatric Home Care: An Institutionally Based Outreach Program." In R. E. K Stein (Ed.), *Caring for Children with Chronic Illness* (pp. 161–72). New York: Springer-Verlag.

Aday, L. A., Aitken, M. J., & Wegener, D. H. (1988). *Pediatric Home Care: Results of a National Evaluation of Programs for Ventilator Assisted Children.* Chicago: Pluribus Press.

Aledort, L., et al. (1988). "Hemophilia—A Treatment in Crisis." *New England Journal of Medicine, 319,* 1017.

American Academy of Pediatrics, Committee on Children with Disabilities (1986). "Transition of Severely Disabled Children from Hospital or Chronic Care Facility to the Community." *Pediatrics, 78,* 531–34.

American Academy of Pediatrics (1987). "Health Care Financing for the Child with Catastrophic Costs." *Pediatrics, 80,* 752–57.

Anderson, B. (1985, Winter–Spring). "Parents of Children with Disabilities as Collaborators in Home Health Care." *Coalition Quarterly, 4*(2, 3), 1–18. Publication of Federation for Children with Special Needs, 312 Stuart St., Boston, MA 02116.

Anderson, J. M., & Elfert, H. (1989). "Managing Chronic Stress in the Family: Women as Caretakers." *Journal of Advanced Nursing, 14,* 735–43.

Applebaum, R., & Christianson, J. (1988, July). "Using Case Management to Monitor Community-Based Long Term Care." *Quality Review Bulletin,* 227–31.

Association for the Care of Children's Health (1984). *Home Care for Children with Serious Handicapping Conditions.* Conference report.

Baird, S. M., & Ashcroft, S. C. (1985). "Need-Based Educational Policy for Chronically Ill Children." In N. Hobbs & J. M. Perrin (Eds.), *Issues in the Care of Children with Chronic Illness: A Sourcebook on Problems, Services, and Policies* (pp. 656–71). San Francisco: Jossey-Bass.

Banaszak, E., et al. (1981). "Home Ventilator Care." *Respiratory Care, 26,* 1262–68.

Bauchner, H., Brown, E., & Peskin, J. (1988). "Premature Graduates of the Neonatal Intensive Care Unit: A Guide to Follow-up." *Pediatric Clinics of North America, 35,* 1207–26.

Bilotti, G. E. (1989). "The Illinois Model: A Statewide Initiative." In R. E. K. Stein (Ed.), *Caring for Children with Chronic Illness* (pp. 185–95). New York: Springer-Verlag.

Blagg, C. R., et al. (1970). "Home Hemodialysis: Six Years' Experience." *New England Journal of Medicine, 283*, 1126–31.

Bloom, B., et al. (1985). "The Epidemiology of Disease Expenses." *Journal of the American Medical Association, 253*, 2393–97.

Blumstein, J. F. (1988). "Effective Health Planning in a Competitive Environment." In F. A. Sloan, J. F. Blumstein, & J. M. Perrin (Eds.), *Cost, Quality, and Access in Health Care* (pp. 21–43). San Francisco: Jossey-Bass.

Bock, R. H., et al. (1983). "There's No Place Like Home." *Children's Health Care, 12*, 93–95.

Branch, L. G., et al. (1988). "A Prospective Study of Incident Comprehensive Medical Home Care Use Among the Elderly." *American Journal of Public Health, 78*, 255–59.

Breslau, N. (1983). "Care of Disabled Children and Women's Time Use." *Medical Care, 21*, 620–29.

Breslau, N. (1985). "Psychiatric Disorder in Children with Physical Disabilities." *Journal of the American Academy of Child Psychiatry, 24*, 87–94.

Breslau, N., & Davis, G. C. (1986). "Chronic Stress and Major Depression." *Archives of General Psychiatry, 43*, 309–14.

Breslau, N., & Marshall, I. A. (1985). "Psychological Disturbance in Children with Physical Disabilities: Continuity and Change in a 5-Year Follow-Up." *Journal of Abnormal Child Psychology, 13*, 199–216.

Breslau, N., & Mortimer, E. A. (1981). "Seeing the Same Doctor: Determinants of Satisfaction with Specialty Care for Disabled Children." *Medical Care, 19*, 741–58.

Breslau, N., Salkever, D., & Staruch K. (1982). "Women's Labor Force Activity and Responsibilities for Disabled Dependents: A Study of Families with Disabled Children." *Journal of Health and Social Behavior, 23*, 169–83.

Brimblecombe, F. S. W. (1974). "Exeter Project for Handicapped Children." *British Medical Journal, 4*, 706–9.

Brody, J. (1991, October 1). "A Quality of Life Determined by a Baby's Size." *New York Times* (national ed.), p. A1.

Burr, B. H., et al. (1983). "Home Care for Children on Respirators." *New England Journal of Medicine, 309*, 1319–23.

Burr, C. K. (1985). "Impact on the Family of a Chronically Ill Child." In N. Hobbs & J. M. Perrin (Eds.), *Issues in the Care of Children with Chronic Illness* (pp. 24–40). San Francisco: Jossey-Bass.

Butler, J. A., et al. (1985). "Health Care Expenditures for Children with Chronic Illnesses." In N. Hobbs & J. M. Perrin (Eds.), *Issues in the Care of Children with Chronic Illnesses* (pp. 827–63). San Francisco: Jossey-Bass.

Butler, J. A., Winter, W. D., Singer, J. D., & Wenger, M. (1985b). "Medical Care

Use and Expenditures Among Children and Youth in the United States: Analysis of a National Probability Sample." *Pediatrics*, *76*, 495–507.

Cadman, D., Boyle, M., Szatmari, P., & Offord, D. R. (1987). "Chronic Illness, Disability, and Mental and Social Well-being." *Pediatrics*, *79*, 805–13.

Campbell, J., & Campbell, A. (1978). "The Social and Economic Costs of End-Stage Renal Disease." *New England Journal of Medicine*, *299*, 386–92.

Carpenter, E. (1980). "Children's Health Care and the Changing Role of Women." *Medical Care*, *18*, 1208–18.

Case, J., & Matthews, S. (1983). "CHIP: The Chronic Health Impaired Program of the Baltimore City Public School System." *Children's Health Care*, *12*, 97–99.

Centers for Disease Control (1989). "Economic Burden of Spina Bifida—United States, 1980–1990." *Morbidity and Mortality Weekly Report*, *38*, 264–67.

Child Health in 1990: The U.S. compared to Canada, England and Wales, France, the Netherlands, and Norway. *Pediatrics, 86* (Suppl.) 1025–1127.

Committee for Economic Development (1987). *Children in Need: Investment Strategies for the Educationally Disadvantaged.* New York: Author.

Counts, S., et al. (1973). "Chronic Home Peritoneal Dialysis in Children." *Transactions of the American Society of Artificial Organs*, *19*, 157–63.

Cystic Fibrosis Foundation (1980). "Cost of CF Survey: Summary of Results."

Davies, A. R., & Ware, J. E. (1988). "Involving Consumers in Quality of Care Assessment." *Health Affairs*, *7*, 33–48.

Delano, B. G., et al. (1981). "Home and Medical Center Hemodialysis: Dollar Comparison and Payback Period." *Journal of the American Medical Association*, *246*, 230–32.

Detsel v. Sullivan, 895 F.2d 58 (2d Cir. 1990).

Donabedian, A. (1980). *Explorations in Quality Assessment and Monitoring: Vol. 1. The Definition of Quality and Approaches to its Assessment*, Ann Arbor, MI: Health Administration Press.

Donabedian, A. (1989). "The End Results of Health Care: Ernest Codman's Contribution to Quality Assessment and Beyond." *The Milbank Quarterly*, *67*, 233–56.

Donati, M. A., Guenette, G., & Auerbach, H. (1987). "Prospective Controlled Study of Home and Hospital Therapy of Cystic Fibrosis Pulmonary Disease." *Journal of Pediatrics*, *111*, 28–33.

Donn, S. (1982). "Cost-Effectiveness of Home Management of Bronchopulmonary Dysplasia." *Pediatrics*, *70*, 330–31.

Edwardson, S. R. (1983). "The Choice Between Hospital and Home Care for Terminally Ill Children." *Nursing Research*, *32*, 29–34.

Edwardson, S. R. (1985). "Physician Acceptance of Home Care of Terminally Ill Children." *Health Services Research*, *20*, 83–100.

Enthoven, A., & Kronick, R. (1989). "A Consumer-Choice Health Plan for the 1990s." *New England Journal of Medicine*, *320*, 29–37.

Farley, P. (1985). "Who Are the Underinsured?" *Milbank Memorial Fund Quarterly*, *63*, 476–503.

Feinberg, E. A. (1985, May). "Family Stress in Pediatric Home Care." *Caring*, *4*(5), 38–44.

Fergusson, J., & Hobbie, W. (1985). "Home Visits for the Child with Cancer." *Nursing Clinics of North America, 20*, 109–15.

Foster, J., & Hoskins, D. (1981). "Home Care of the Child with a Tracheotomy Tube." *Pediatric Clinics of North America, 28*, 855–57.

Fox, H. (1984, September). "A Preliminary Analysis of Options to Improve Health Insurance Coverage for Chronically Ill and Disabled Children." Report prepared for the U.S. Department of Health and Human Services, Division of Maternal and Child Health, Habilitative Services Branch.

Fox, H. B. (1990, January 12). "1989 Legislative Amendments Affecting Access to Care by Children and Pregnant Women." Memorandum to the state directors of Maternal and Child Health Services and Programs for Children with Special Health Care Needs and Other Interested Persons. Washington, D.C.: Fox Health Policy Consultants.

Fox, H. B., & Greaney, A. (1988, December). "Disabled Children's Access to Supplemental Security Income and Medicaid Benefits." Prepared for the University of California at San Francisco with support from the U.S. Department of Health and Human Services, Bureau of Maternal and Child Health and Resources Development. Washington, D.C.: Fox Health Policy Consultants.

Fox, H. B., & Newacheck, P. (1990). "Private Health Insurance of Chronically Ill Children." *Pediatrics, 85*, 50–57.

Fox, H. B., et al. (1987, December 14–15). "Briefing Memoranda for Meeting on the Feasibility of High-Risk Pools to Provide Health Insurance Protection for Children with Special Health Care Needs." Washington, D.C.: Fox Health Policy Consultants.

Fox, H. B., et al. (1990, September). "An Examination of HMO Policies Affecting Children with Special Needs." Washington D.C.: Fox Health Policy Consultants.

Frates, R. C., et al. (1985). "Outcome of Home Mechanical Ventilation in Children." *Journal of Pediatrics, 106*, 850–56.

Freedman, S. A., & Pierce, P. M. (1989). "REACH: A Rural Case-Management Project." In R. E. K. Stein (Ed.), *Caring for Children with Chronic Illness* (pp. 173–84). New York: Springer-Verlag.

General Accounting Office (1986, December). *Medicare: Need to Strengthen Home Health Care Payment Controls and Address Unmet Needs* (GAO/HRD–87–9). Washington DC: U.S. Government Printing Office.

General Accounting Office (1989). "Home Care Experiences of Families with Chronically Ill Children" (Report No. GAO/HRD-89–73). Gaithersburg, Md: U.S. Government Printing Office.

Ginsburg, J. A., & the Health and Public Policy Committee, American College of

Physicians (1986). "Home Health Care." *Annals of Internal Medicine*, *105*, 454–60.

Gittler, J., & Colton, M. (1986). "Community-Based Case Management Programs for Children with Special Health Care Needs." Maternal and Child Health Resource Center, Iowa City, IA.

Goldberg, A. I., et al. (1984). "Home Care for Life-Supported Persons: An Approach to Program Development." *Journal of Pediatrics*, *104*, 785–95.

Goldberg, M., Baugham, K., & Wombolt, D. (1980). "Home Intermittent Peritoneal Dialysis." *Proceedings from Clinical Dialysis and Transplant Forum*, *10*, 224–26.

Goodwin, S. (1990). "Children with Special Needs in England and Wales." *Pediatrics*, *86*, 1112–16.

Gorham, W., & Glazer, N. (1976). *The Urban Predicament*. Washington, D.C.: The Urban Institute.

Gortmaker, S. L. (1985). "Demography of Chronic Childhood Diseases." In N. Hobbs & J. M. Perrin (Eds.), *Issues in the Care of Children with Chronic Illnesses* (pp. 134–54). San Francisco: Jossey-Bass.

Gortmaker, S., & Sappenfield, W. (1984). "Chronic Childhood Disorders: Prevalence and Impact." *Pediatric Clinics of North America*, *31*, 3–18.

Gurdin, P., & Anderson, G. R. (1991). "Specialized Foster Care for Children with HIV." In N. J. Hochstadt & D. M. Yost (Eds.), *The Medically Complex Child: The Transition to Home Care* (pp. 219–28). Chur, Switzerland: Harwood Academic Publishers.

Hall, L. (1990). "Medicaid Home Care Options for Disabled Children." Health Policy Department, Human Resources Policy Studies Division, Center for Policy Research, National Governors Association, Washington, DC.

Hippolitus, P. (1985). "Employment Opportunities and Services for Youth with Chronic Illnesses." In N. Hobbs & J. M. Perrin (Eds.), *Issues in the Care of Children with Chronic Illnesses* (pp. 716–30). San Francisco: Jossey-Bass.

Hobbs, N., Perrin, J. M., & Ireys, H. T. (1985). *Chronically Ill Children and Their Families*. San Francisco: Jossey-Bass.

Hochstadt, N. J., & Yost, D. M. (Eds.) (1991). *The Medically Complex Child: The Transition to Home Care*. Chur, Switzerland: Harwood Academic Publishers.

Hoffman, E. L., & Bennett, F. C. (1990). "Birthweight Less Than 800 Grams: Changing Outcomes and Influences of Gender and Gestation Number." *Pediatrics*, *86*, 27–34.

Hoffstein, P., et al. (1976). "Dialysis Costs: Results of a Diverse Sample Study." *Kidney International*, *9*, 286–93.

Holmes, G., et al. (1986). "The Availability of Insurance to Long-Time Survivors of Childhood Cancer." *Cancer*, *57*, 190–93.

Holtzman, N. A., & Richmond, J. (1985). "Genetic Strategies for Preventing Chronic Illnesses." In N. Hobbs & J. M. Perrin (Eds.), *Issues in the Care of Children with Chronic Illness* (pp. 87–108). San Francisco: Jossey-Bass.

Infant Health and Development Program (1990). "Enhancing the Outcomes of Low Birth Weight, Premature Infants: A Multi-site Randomized Trial." *Journal of the American Medical Association, 263*, 303–42.

Institute of Medicine (1991). *Disability in America: Toward a National Agenda for Prevention*. Washington D.C.: National Academy Press.

Ireys, H. T. (1981). "Health Care for Chronically Disabled Children and their Families." In *Better Health for Our Children: A National Strategy. The Report of the Select Panel for the Promotion of Child Health: Vol. IV*. Washington, D.C.: U.S. Government Printing Office.

Ireys, H., & Eichler, R. (1988). "Correlates of Variation Among State Programs for Children with Special Health Care Needs: Report of a Survey and Six Case Studies" (MCJ-360479). Springfield, VA: National Technical Information Service, U.S. Department of Commerce.

Ireys, H. T., Hauck, R. J. P., & Perrin, J. M. "Variability Among State Crippled Children's Service Programs: Pluralism Thrives." *American Journal of Public Health, 75*, 375–81.

Jessop, D. J., & Stein, R. E. K. (1985). "Uncertainty and Its Relation to the Psychological and Social Correlates of Chronic Illness in Children." *Social Science and Medicine, 20*, 993–99.

Kacmarek, R. M., & Thompson, J. E. (1986). "Respiratory Care of the Ventilator-Assisted Infant in the Home." *Respiratory Care, 31*, 605–14.

Kane, R. L. (1991, April 8–9). "The Implications for Quality Assurance of the Move to More Community-Based Care." Report prepared for the Institute of Medicine Meeting on Quality of Care Implications of Shift in Care to Home and Community Settings.

Kanthor, H., et al. (1974). "Areas of Responsibility in the Health Care of Multiply Handicapped Children." *Pediatrics, 54*, 779–88.

Kaufert, J. M. (1980). "Social and Psychological Responses to Home Therapy of Hemophilia." *Journal of Epidemiology and Community Health, 34*, 194–200.

Kinzer, D. M. (1990). "Universal Entitlement to Health Care." *New England Journal of Medicine, 322*, 467–70.

Klerman, L. (1985). "Interpersonal Issues in Delivering Services to Chronically Ill Children and Their Families." In N. Hobbs & J. M. Perrin (Eds.), *Issues in the Care of Children with Chronic Illness* (pp. 420–40). San Francisco: Jossey-Bass.

Kopelman, L. "Paternalism and Autonomy in the Care of Chronically Ill Children." In N. Hobbs & J. M. Perrin (Eds.), *Issues in the Care of Children with Chronic Illness* (pp. 61–86). San Francisco: Jossey-Bass.

Koren, M. J. (1986). "Home Care—Who Cares?" *New England Journal of Medicine, 314*, 917–20.

Kramer, A. M., Shaughnessy, P. W., Bauman, M. K., & Crisler, K. S. (1990). "Assessing and Assuring the Quality of Home Health Care: A Conceptual Framework." *The Milbank Quarterly, 68*, 413–43.

La Jolla Management Corporation (1986, April). "Financing Care of Chronically Ill and Disabled Children in Home and Other Ambulatory Care Settings.'' Report to the Department of Health and Human Services, Division of Maternal and Child Health, Rockville, MD.

Lansky, S., et al. (1979). ''Childhood Cancer: Nonmedical Costs of the Illness.'' *Cancer, 43*, 403–8.

Laudicina, S. (1988). ''State Health Risk Pools: Insuring the 'Uninsurable'.'' *Health Affairs, 7,* 97–104

Lauer, M. E., et al. (1983). ''A Comparison Study of Parental Adaptation Following a Child's Death at Home or in the Hospital.'' *Pediatrics, 71*, 107–12.

Lauer, M. E., et al. (1985, February). ''Children's Perceptions of Their Siblings' Death at Home or in Hospital: The Precursors of Differential Adjustment.'' *Cancer Nursing,* 21–27.

LeQuesne, B., et al. (1974). ''Home Therapy for Patients with Hemophilia.'' *Lancet, 2,* 507–10.

Lewis, I. J., & Sheps, C. G. (1983). *The Sick Citadel,* Cambridge, MA: Oelge-schlager, Gunn, and Hain.

Lie, S. O. (1990). ''Children in the Norwegian Health Care System.'' *Pediatrics, 86,* 1048–52.

Ludman, L., Lansdown, R., & Spitz, L. (1989). ''Factors Associated with Developmental Progress of Full Term Neonates Who Require Intensive Care.'' *Archives of Diseases of Childhood, 64,* 733–37.

MacQueen, J. (1986). ''Iowa's Mobile and Regional Clinics.'' Iowa City: Iowa Department of Public Health.

Magrab, P. R. (1985). ''Psychosocial Development of Chronically Ill Children.'' In N. Hobbs & J. M. Perrin (Eds.), *Issues in the Care of Children with Chronic Illness* (pp. 698–715). San Francisco: Jossey-Bass.

Manton, K. G. (1989). ''Epidemiological, Demographic, and Social Correlates of Disability among the Elderly.'' *Milbank Quarterly, 67* (Suppl. 2), 13–58.

Martin, R. C. ''Legal Issues and Interpretation of P.L. 94–142.'' *Coalition Quarterly.*

Massie, R., & Massie, S. (1976). *Journey.* New York: Knopf.

McCollum, A. (1971). ''Cystic Fibrosis: Economic Impact Upon the Family.'' *American Journal of Public Health, 61,* 1335–40.

McCormick, M., et al. (1986). ''The Impact of Childhood Rheumatic Diseases on the Family.'' *Arthritis and Rheumatism, 29,* 872–79.

McGeary, M. G. H., & Lynn, L. E., Jr. (Eds.). (1988). *Urban Change and Poverty.* Washington, DC: National Academy Press.

McKenzie, L. L., Fie, R., & Van Eys, J. (1974). ''Medical, Economic, and Social Impact of a Home Therapy Program for Hemophilia A on Selected Patients.'' *Southern Medical Journal, 67,* 555–59.

McLanahan, S., & Adams, J. (1987). ''Parenthood and Psychological Well-Being.'' *Annual Review of Sociology, 13,* 237–257.

McLaughlin, J., & Shurtleff, D. (1979). ''Management of the Newborn with Myelodysplasia.'' *Clinical Pediatrics, 18,* 463–76.

McManus, M. (1989, January). *A Statistical Profile of Children and Pregnant*

Women. American Academy of Pediatrics, Congressional Health Policy Retreat.

McManus, M., & Greaney, A. (1988, Fall). "Health Insurance Snapshot of Children: A Crisis Situation." American Academy of Pediatrics Child Health Financing Report.

Mearig, J. S. (1985). "Cognitive Development of Chronically Ill Children." In N. Hobbs & J. M. Perrin (Eds.), *Issues in the Care of Children with Chronic Illness* (pp. 672–97). San Francisco: Jossey-Bass.

Meisels, S. J., & Shonkoff, J. P. (Eds.). *Handbook of Early Childhood Intervention.* New York: Cambridge University Press.

Merkens, M. J. (1991). "From Intensive Care Unit to Home: The Role of Pediatric Transitional Care." In N. J. Hochstadt & D. M. Yost (Eds.), *The Medically Complex Child: The Transition to Home Care* (pp. 61–78). Chur, Switzerland: Harwood Academic Publishers.

Moldow, D. G., & Martinson, I. M. (1980). "From Research to Reality—Home Care for the Dying Child." *Maternal and Child Nursing, 5,* 159–66.

Moldow, D. G., et al. (1982). "The Cost of Home Care for Dying Children." *Medical Care, 20,* 1154–60.

Mor, V., Wachtel, T. J., & Kidder, D. (1985). "Patient Predictors of Hospice Use." *Medical Care, 23,* 1115–19.

National Hemophilia Foundation Bulletins: Supply Watch Bulletins No. 11 (November 21, 1988, and update of December 5, 1988) and No. 16 (May 19, 1989). Finance and Reimbursement Bulletins No. 23 (April 23, 1990) and No. 26 (February 1991).

New England SERVE. (1989). *Enhancing Quality.* Boston: New England SERVE.

Newacheck, P. (1988). "Estimating Medicaid-Eligible Pregnant Women and Children Living Below 185% of Poverty." National Governors' Association, Center for Policy Research.

Newacheck, P. W., Budetti, P. P., & McManus, P. (1984). "Trends in Childhood Disability." *American Journal of Public Health, 74,* 232–36.

Newacheck, P., & McManus, M. (1988). "Financing Health Care for Disabled Children." *Pediatrics, 81,* 385–94.

Newton, L., et al. (1982). "Home Care of the Pediatric Patient with a Tracheotomy." *Annals of Otology Rhinology and Laryngology, 91,* 633–40.

Okamoto, G., & Shurtleff, D. A. (1981). "Perceived First Contact Care for Disabled Children." *Pediatrics, 67,* 530–35.

Oppenheimer, J. R., & Rucker, R. W. (1980). "The Effect of Parental Relationships on the Management of Cystic Fibrosis and Guidelines for Social Work Intervention." *Social Work in Health Care, 5,* 409–19.

Oster, A. R. (1985, Winter–Spring). "Parents and Professionals: the Essential Partnership for Families in Crisis." *Coalition Quarterly, 4*(2, 3), 5–8. Publication of Federation for Children with Special Needs, 312 Stuart St., Boston, MA 02116.

Outka, G. (1975). "Social Justice and Equal Access to Health Care." *Perspectives in Biology and Medicine, 18,* 185–203.

Pear, R. (1988, March 6). "Expanded Right to Medicaid Shatters the Link to Welfare." *New York Times*, p. 1.

Perrin, E. C., Stein, R. E., & Drotar, D. (1991). "Cautions in Using the Child Behavior Checklist: Observations Based on Research about Children with a Chronic Illness." *Journal of Pediatric Psychology*, *16*, 411–21.

Perrin, J. M. (1990). "Children with Special Health Needs: A U.S. Perspective." *Pediatrics*, *86*, 1120–23.

Perrin, J. M., & Stein, R. E. K. (1991). "Reinterpreting Disability: Changes in SSI for Children." *Pediatrics*, *88*, 1047–51.

Pierce, P. M., & Freedman, S. A. (1983). "The REACH Program: An Innovative Delivery Model for Medically Dependent Children." *Children's Health Care*, *12*, 86–89.

Pierce, P. M., Lester, D. G., & Fraze, D. E. (1991). "Prescribed Pediatric Extended Care: The Family Centered Health Care Alternative for Medically and Technology Dependent Children. In N. J. Hochstadt & D. M. Yost (Eds.), *The Medically Complex Child: The Transition to Home Care* (pp. 177–90). Chur, Switzerland: Harwood Academic Publishers.

Pless, I. B., & Pinkerton, P. (1975). *Chronic Childhood Disorder: Promoting Patterns of Adjustment*. Chicago: Year Book Medical Publishers.

Pless, I. B., & Roghmann, K. J. (1971). "Chronic Illness and Its Consequences: Observations Based on Three Epidemiologic Surveys." *Journal of Pediatrics*, *79*, 351–59.

Pless, I. B., & Satterwhite, B. B. (1972). "Chronic Illness in Children: Selection, Activities, and Evaluation of Non-Professional Family Counselors." *Clinical Pediatrics*, *11*, 403–10.

Pless, I. B., Satterwhite, B., & Van Vechten, D. (1978). "Division, Duplication, and Neglect: Patterns of Care for Children with Chronic Disorders." *Child*, *4*, 9–19.

Prentice, W. S. (1986). "Placement Alternatives for Long-Term Ventilator Care." *Respiratory Care*, *31*, 288–93.

Prybyl, L., & Prybyl, T. (1991). "Medical Foster Care: The Foster Parents' Perspective." In N. J. Hochstadt & D. M. Yost (Eds.), *The Medically Complex Child: The Transition to Home Care* (pp. 139–52). Chur, Switzerland: Harwood Academic Publishers.

Quint, R., et al. (1990). "Home Care for Ventilator-Dependent Children: Psychosocial Impact on the Family." *American Journal of Diseases of Children*, *144*, 1238–41.

Rieser, L. (1986). "Educational Rights of Children with Health Impairments." In D. K. Walker (Ed.), *School-Age Children with Health Impairments* Boston, MA: Harvard School of Public Health.

Robinovitch, A. (1981). "Home Total Parenteral Nutrition: A Psychological Viewpoint." *Journal of Parenteral and Enteral Nutrition*. *5*, 522–25.

Rosenbaum, S. (1988, May). Testimony of the Children's Defense Fund Before the Senate Finance Committee.

Ruben, R. J., et al. (1982, November–December). "Home Care of the Pediatric

Patient with a Tracheotomy.'' *Annals of Otology, Rhinology and Laryngology*, *91*, 633–40.

Rucker, R. W., & Harrison, G. M. (1974). ''Outpatient Intravenous Medications in the Management of Cystic Fibrosis.'' *Pediatrics*, *54*, 358–60.

Salkever, D. (1982). ''Communications: Children's Health Problems and Maternal Work Status.'' *Journal of Human Resources*, *17*, 94–109.

Samuelson, P., & Nordhaus, W. (1989). *Economics*. New York: McGraw-Hill.

Shayne, M. W., Walker, D. K., Perrin, J. M., & Moynihan, L. C. (1987). ''Health-Impaired Children Deserve a Break.'' *Principal*, *66*, 36–39.

Shurtleff, D., et al. (1974). ''Myelodysplasia: Decision for Death or Disability.'' *New England Journal of Medicine*, *291*, 1005–11.

Singer, J. D., & Butler, J. A. (1987). ''The Education for All Handicapped Children Act: Schools as Agents of Social Reform.'' *Harvard Educational Review*, *57*, 125–52.

Sivak, E., et al. (1983). ''Pulmonary Mechanical Ventilation at Home: A Reasonable and Less Expensive Alternative.'' *Respiratory Care*, *28*, 42–49.

Sloan, F. A., Blumstein, J. F., & Perrin, J. M. (Eds.). (1988). *Cost, Quality, and Access in Health Care*. San Francisco: Jossey-Bass.

Smith, P. S., & Levine, P. (1984). ''The Benefits of Comprehensive Care of Hemophilia: A Five-Year Study of Outcomes.'' *American Journal of Public Health*, *74*, 616–17.

Smyth-Staruch, K., et al. (1984). ''Use of Health Services by Chronically Ill and Disabled Children.'' *Medical Care*, *22*, 310–28.

Stein, R. E. K. (1985). ''Home Care: A Challenging Opportunity.'' *Children's Health Care*, *14*, 90–95.

Stein, R. E. K. (1987, January). ''Providing Home Care for the Seriously Ill Young.'' *Business and Health*, *4*, 22–29.

Stein, R. E. K. (Ed.). (1989). *Caring for Children with Chronic Illness*. New York: Springer-Verlag.

Stein, R. E. K., & Jessop, D. J. (1984). *Evaluation of a Home Care Unit as an Ambulatory ICU*. Springfield, VA: National Technical Information Service.

Stein, R. E. K., & Jessop, D. J. (1985). ''Delivery of Care to Inner-City Children with Chronic Conditions.'' In N. Hobbs & J. M. Perrin (Eds.), *Issues in the Care of Children with Chronic Illness* (pp. 382–401). San Francisco: Jossey-Bass.

Stein, R. E. K., & Jessop, D. J. (1990). ''Functional Status II(R).'' *Medical Care*, *28*, 1041–55.

Stein, R. E. K., & Riessman, C. (1980). ''The Development of an Impact-on-Family Scale: Preliminary Findings.'' *Medical Care*, *18*, 465–72.

Stiver, H., et al. (1982). ''Self-Administration of Intravenous Antibiotics: An Efficient, Cost-Effective Home Care Program.'' *Canadian Medical Association Journal*, *127*, 207–11.

Strawczynski, H., et al. (1973). ''Delivery of Care to Hemophiliac Children: Home Care vs. Hospitalization.'' *Pediatrics*, *51*, 986–91.

Strayer, F., Kisker, C. T., & Fethke, C. (1990). ''Cost-Effectiveness of a Shared-

Management Delivery System for the Care of Children with Cancer." *Pediatrics, 66*, 907–11.

Sullivan v. Zebley, 110 S. Ct. 885 (1990).

Tarlov, A. R., Ware, J. E., Greenfield, S., Nelson, E. C., Perrin, E., & Zubkoff, M. (1989). "The Medical Outcomes Study: An Application of Methods for Monitoring the Results of Medical Care." *Journal of the American Medical Association, 262*, 925–30.

Thorp, E. K. (1987, May). "Mothers' Coping with Home Care of Severe Chronic Respiratory Disabled Children Requiring Medical Technology Assistance." Dissertation submitted to the faculty of the School of Education and Development, George Washington University, Washington, DC.

Turner-Henson, A., Swan, J. H., & Holaday, B. (1991, November). "Friendship Patterns and Activities in Chronically Ill Children." Paper presented at the annual meeting of the American Public Health Association, Atlanta.

U.S. Congress (1983). Education of the Handicapped Act, Section 618, as amended by Public Law 98–199.

U.S. Congress (1987). Office of Technology Assessment, "Technology Dependent Children: Hospital v. Home Care—A Technical Memorandum" (OTA-TM-H-38). Washington, D.C.: U.S. Government Printing Office.

U.S. Department of Education (1987). Office of Special Education and Rehabilitative Services. "Ninth Annual Report to Congress on the Implementation of The Education of the Handicapped Act." Prepared by the Division of Innovation and Development, Office of Special Education Programs.

U.S. Department of Education (1990). Office of Special Education and Rehabilitative Services. "Twelfth Annual Report to Congress on the Implementation of The Education of the Handicapped Act." Prepared by the Division of Innovation and Development, Office of Special Education Programs.

U.S. Department of Health and Human Services (1982, December 13–14). *Report of the Surgeon General's Workshop on Children With Handicaps and their Families*. Washington, D.C.: Author.

U.S. Department of Health and Human Services (1987). Health Care Financing Administration, Office of the Actuary. *Health Care Financing, Program Statistics, Analysis of State Medicaid Program Characteristics, 1986* (HCFA Pub. No. 03249).

U.S. Department of Health and Human Services (1988, April 7). *Fostering Home and Community-Based Care for Technology-Dependent Children* (Vol. 2). (HCFA Pub. No. 88–02171). Washington, D.C.: Author.

U.S. Department of Health and Human Services (1989). Health Care Financing Administration, Office of Research and Demonstrations. *Health Care Financing, Program Statistics, Medicare and Medicaid Data Book, 1988* (HCFA Pub. No. 03270).

U.S. Department of Health and Human Services (1990). *Healthy People 2000: National Health Promotion and Disease Prevention Objectives* (DHHS Pub. No [PHS] 91–50213). Washington, D.C.: U.S. Government Printing Office.

U.S. Department of Labor, Bureau of Labor Statistics (1990). "Consumer Price Indexes, Major Expenditure Classes, 1946–89." In *Economic Report to the President Transmitted to Congress,* February 1990, p. 359, Table C-58. Washington, D.C.: U.S. Government Printing Office.

Walker, D. K., Stein, R. E. K., Perrin, E. C., & Jessop, D. J. (1990). "Assessing Psychosocial Adjustment of Children with Chronic Illnesses: A Review of the Technical Properties of PARS III." *Journal of Developmental and Behavioral Pediatrics, 11,* 116–21.

Walker, D. K. (Ed.). (1986, January). "Report of a National Conference: School-Age Children with Health Impairments." Mimeograph, Boston.

Weeks, K. (1985). "Private Health Insurance and Chronically Ill Children." In N. Hobbs & J. M. Perrin (Eds.), *Issues in the Care of Children with Chronic Illness* (pp. 880–911). San Francisco: Jossey-Bass.

Wilensky, G. (1988). "Filling the Gaps in Health Insurance: Impact on Competition." *Health Affairs, 7,* 133–49.

Wilson, W. J. (1987). *The Truly Disadvantaged: The Inner-City, The Underclass, and Public Policy.* Chicago: University of Chicago Press.

Index